# REIKI HEALING FOR BEGINNERS

The Complete Beginner's Guide to Reiki Healing. Balance and Increase Your Energy, Relieve Stress

BY

Deepali Nara

The information herein is offered for informational purposes solely, and is universal as so. The presentation of the information is without contract or any type of guarantee assurance.

The trademarks that are used are without any consent, and the publication of the trademark is without permission or backing by the trademark owner. All trademarks and brands within this book are for clarifying purposes only and are the owned by the owners themselves, not affiliated with this document.

# Disclaimer

All erudition contained in this book is given for informational and educational purposes only. The author is not in any way accountable for any results or outcomes that emanate from using this material. Constructive attempts have been made to provide information that is both accurate and effective, but the author is not bound for the accuracy or use/misuse of this information.

# Foreword

First, I will like to thank you for taking the first step of trusting me and deciding to purchase/read this life-transforming eBook. Thanks for spending your time and resources on this material.

I can assure you of exact results if you will diligently follow the exact blueprint, I lay bare in the information manual you are currently reading. It has transformed lives, and I strongly believe it will equally transform your own life too.

All the information I presented in this Do It Yourself piece is easy to digest and practice.

# CONTENTS

# INTRODUCTION

Reiki, the recuperating treatment made by a Japanese Buddhist named Mikao Usui over a hundred years prior, depends on a basic otherworldly standard: We're altogether guided by the equivalent imperceptible life power, and it controls our physical, mental, and enthusiastic prosperity. At the point when the vitality streams unreservedly, we can take advantage of obscure stores of intensity. When it keeps running into blockages (frequently said to be brought about by negative reasoning, unhealed injury, or stress over-burden), we work at an imperfect level.

The story goes like this-Dr. Usui had been to the highest point of Mt. Kurama in Japan in the year 1922 on a three-week trip. While reflecting at Mt. Kurama, he had a dream on the 21st day where he has decreed as a healer himself in an antiquated mending framework. On his way back to his home, he could understand he was in a situation to recuperate wounds of individuals incorporating his very own with astounding flawlessness and speed.

While this may seem like voodoo enchantment to a few, even nonbelievers who have gone through an hour with a gifted Reiki ace (as they're called) have felt a positive move or the like. Many portray Reiki sessions—a blend of light touch or more the-body vitality clearing—as quieting or establishing. Furthermore, for other people, it feels progressively like an enthusiastic realignment.

From there on, he started a center in Tokyo and treated numerous patients. He likewise prepared numerous individuals to be Reiki professionals. After the staggering tremor in Kanto in the year 1923, Reiki as a type of recuperating workmanship had demonstrated its value. For his mending administration, Dr. Usui was granted by the Japanese government. During the 1930s a Hawaiian lady of Japanese starting point named Hawayo Takata created Reiki in the United States. Takata herself increased extraordinary advantage for her medical issues by virtue of Reiki application.

After her own recuperating knowledge, she started to learn, practice, and afterward instruct Reiki in Hawaii. She conferred Reiki for quite a while until her passing in 1980. From that point, Reiki spread to different nations where Reiki centers and Reiki Masters had their influence to give recuperating contact to different sicknesses through this antiquated framework. Inevitably, Reiki has picked up acknowledgment, acknowledgment and noticeable quality being an antiquated type of recuperating system. In spite of the fact that the Reiki medications offered nowadays are a bit not quite the same as the old ones, yet they are essentially they have a place with a similar type of recuperating vitality of Reiki.

Reiki embraces the procedure of vitality mending for pressure unwinding and decrease. Regardless of the headway of therapeutic sciences, Reiki is in effect, progressively utilized as a corresponding treatment to determine different medical issues. In Reiki, everything is a supernatural occurrence in light of the fact that in this type of treatment, all-encompassing, impalpable, undetectable fragile type of vitality is grinding away. Reiki utilizes the vitality to advance agreement in living things that encourages the mending of the psyche, body, and soul. In short, Reiki recuperates at the physical, passionate, and profound degree of a person.

With an expanded degree of mindfulness among masses, individuals began expecting suppliers of social insurance give benefits through various normal recuperating procedures, including Reiki. Keeping in view the requests of the patients requiring normal social insurance benefits, the notoriety of Reiki has been developing step by step with its expanded use of Reiki in different centers and emergency clinics. Beginning Reiki preparing projects are currently being bestowed in Hospitals. These classes encourage in setting up the doctors, attendants, and other therapeutic experts to utilize this common recuperating system while interfacing with patients.

A few emergency clinics, Clinics, restorative establishments have been looking into on the adequacy of Reiki Healing. There are more than one hundred offices in the U.S. that utilization Reiki and additionally other corresponding/elective modalities (CAM) in addition to a few hundred increasingly around the world. Furthermore, inquire about is being led in an organization with the National Institutes of Health at a developing number of well-regarded offices. There as of now Reiki programs at Sharp Memorial Hospital - San Diego, St. Joseph Medical Center - Stockton and Hearst Cancer Resource Center - San Luis Obispo to name a not many.

Reiki strategies give recuperating through vitality, diminishes the worry during asymptomatic strategy, controls enthusiastic response to a stunning finding, loosens up the body and mind and improves the nature of rest and quiet down powerless guardians of kids who are truly sick. According to the Reiki, life vitality goes into the Chakra where its necessities for mending vitality are the most. Infants and youngsters regularly get successful outcome as they don't have any psychological barrier in accepting vitality through Reiki. For instance, a crying infant gets speedy solace when he is contacted or grabbed. So also, while managing old individuals in the clinics, in contrast to contacting babies for recuperating, Reiki utilizes two overlap benefits one is giving vitality and unwinding, and the other one is passionate sustenance.

The outcomes coming through such examinations are empowering, and the equivalent has enormously expanded the confidence and dependability of the majority on Reiki as an elective type of treatment. You have to recall the way that the existence of power depends on the vitality, and Reiki theory depends on vitality and vitality as it were. Reiki has gone through a long voyage giving wellbeing and recuperating to its experts and recipients similarly well. Reiki is winding up more broadly acknowledged in the present frameworks of Natural drugs, including Allopathic, Homeopathic, and Acupuncture. We should take cautious note that the utilization of Reiki is imperative as a strengthening if the not integral type of medications and its well-known use will guarantee that Reiki spread out its significance, acknowledgment and noticeable quality as an absolutely real type of common recuperating treatment.

# CHAPTER ONE

## THE SEVEN CHAKRAS

You've presumably heard individuals discussing the seven chakras. They are regularly referenced with regards to enthusiastic mending or contemplation practice. Be that as it may, you may have discovered the idea of chakras confounding. Or on the other hand, you have not exactly comprehended what spot it might have in your life. Things being what they are, everybody can work with chakras, not simply specialists. Every one of these powerful vitality focuses a one of a kind vibrational recurrence. Along these lines, even an essential comprehension of the seven chakras can upgrade your life in astounding ways. Regardless of whether you're attempting to recuperate a particular injury, hoping to improve your appearance work with the Law of Attraction, or simply wanting to support your general prosperity, it pays to find out about the seven chakras. In this current amateur's manual for chakras, we'll investigate each chakra's importance and hues. Moreover, we'll think about how to adjust your seven chakras generally successfully.

## What Is a Chakra?

Chakra means "wheel." The seven chakras in the body are unmistakable vitality focuses that start at the highest point of your head and end at the base of your spine. They direct all pieces of your substantial framework, affecting everything from enthusiastic preparing to protection from sickness. Normally, seven chakras contemplation strategies center around making the chakras open and keeping them in the arrangement. On the off chance that they become shut or out of match up, this can adversely affect your physical and mental wellbeing.

To improve the feeling of how this functions, picture a physical machine. On the off chance that pinions stall out, funnels become withdrawn or parts of the machine spill, it never again carries out its responsibility appropriately. In addition, this essential blame definitely lead to facilitate disappointments. At that point, the gadget falls apart further. The system of chakras works in a comprehensively comparative manner.

When you can tune into the area of your seven chakras, you become proficient at opening chakras and create instincts about blockages. Thusly, you can identify and take care of issues as they emerge, and before they have genuine outcomes. Also, you can find old injuries and take every necessary step expected to address them. In aggregate, through legitimate information of chakras, mending can happen. We'll take a gander at explicit instances of this underneath.

## Chakra History and Traditions

As you expect to address the inquiry "what are the seven chakras?", it's critical to take a gander at the verifiable causes of the seven chakras. The idea follows back to early Hinduism and Buddhism. Hinduism specifically archives up to seven chakras.

Then, Buddhism makes reference to only five. The derivation of the word halfway originates from old Hindu writings, where it is utilized to signify "wheel." It is additionally said to identify with the Greek word "Kuklos," and the Anglo-Saxon word "hveohl." These all assign a wheel or something to that effect. These regular starting points all accentuate the interconnected and continually moving nature of the chakras.

In case no doubt about it "are chakras genuine?", think about that chakra history, unmistakably represents the life span and viability of chakra-based conventions. These real central focuses have been the subject of contemplations, breathing procedures and mantras, all of which means to utilize the chakras to identify, and address, physical and mental issues.

**The Seven Chakras and Where to Locate Them**

Basic chakra activities help you find each chakra, evaluate it, and possibly realign or rebalance it. Strangely, each chakra is additionally connected with a specific component. The seven chakras images and related components can enable you to choose delegate objects for sign work or reflection. Think about this area as a sort of "how to adjust chakras for learners." It will give you the nuts and bolts you have to turn out to be progressively mindful of, and responsible for, this part of yourself, helping you how to unblock your seven chakras when it's required.

## 1. The Root Chakra (Muladhara)

The Root Chakra is fundamental. At the point when everything is great with this chakra, you'll have a sense of safety, quiet and secured in actuality. You'll be strong enough to handle new difficulties, and you'll feel certain doing as such. This makes an appropriately adjusted Root Chakra fundamental at whatever point you're having a go at something new or seeking after a noteworthy all-consuming purpose

You can build up a blocked Root Chakra if something undermines your essential survival needs (for example for sustenance, haven or cash). Regardless of whether you just dread that your essential survival will be undermined, your Root Chakra can leave arrangement accordingly.

- Physical Location: The base of your spine (where your tailbone is found).
- Color: Red.
- Element: Earth.
- Emotional Issues and Behaviors of Blocked Root Chakra: If your Root Chakra is blocked, you may feel compromised, terrified, or on edge. This uneasiness can without much of a stretch penetrate your considerations, making everything all of a sudden vibe unsure. You may likewise find that you can't focus and that you're always distracted with stresses over your prosperity. In certain individuals, this can show as neurosis or general distrustfulness. Physical issues conceivably brought about by a blocked Root Chakra incorporate a sore lower back, low vitality levels, and cold limits.

## 2. The Sacral Chakra (Svadhishthana)

The Sacral Chakra is critical to your innovative vitality. It is connected not exclusively to quest for masterfulness and the creative mind yet in addition to your sexuality and your ability for change in all everyday issues. Your Sacral Chakra may progress toward becoming skewed or obstructed somehow or another in case you're worried about some part of your sexuality. Or then again, on the off chance that you are unsatisfied in your relationship or attempting to encounter joy in life all the more by and large. It can likewise be aggravated by negative criticism that makes you question your innovative limits.

- Physical Location: In the stomach area, approximately two creeps beneath the gut catch.
- Color: Orange.
- Element: Water.
- Emotional Issues and Behaviors of Blocked Sacral Chakra: When there's an issue with the Sacral Chakra, you're probably going to feel exhausted, languid and deadened. You may

have a low sex drive, and you'll conceivably feel scared of (or impervious to) change. Physical manifestations related with a blocked Sacral Chakra can incorporate urinary uneasiness, expanded sensitivities, and a fascination in addictive practices. These need not be identified with medication or liquor use. Shopping fixation, betting, and issues with eating would all be able to be connected to issues with the Sacral Chakra.

### 3. The Solar Plexus Chakra (Manipura)

The Solar Plexus Chakra is frequently thought of as imperative for confidence, self-governance, and assurance. Therefore, it is once in a while called the "individual power" chakra.

At the point when all is as it ought to be with this chakra, you'll have a make way in front of you. You should realize what is fundamental for progress. You may likewise feel autonomous like you can achieve nearly anything on the off chance that you set your focus on it. In the meantime, this chakra can undoubtedly be adversely influenced by seen disappointments, upsetting social encounters, or waiting sentiments of low self-esteem from adolescence.

- Physical Location: Around the stomach zone at the highest point of your belly.
- Color: Yellow.
- Element: Fire.
- Emotional Issues and Behaviors of Blocked Solar Plexus Chakra: If there's a blockage around the Solar Plexus Chakra, your certainty might be extremely flimsy. In the event that there is just a little blockage, there may just be uncertainty in one explicit zone. A bigger blockage can cause summed up confidence issues. You may be spooky by considerations that you are bad enough. Or on the other hand, you may feel incapable of drawing helpful exercises from life's difficulties. Physical challenges related with a blocked Solar Plexus Chakra may incorporate stomach related distress and issues with memory.

## 4. The Heart Chakra (Anahata)

As you may expect, the Heart Chakra is personally associated with your ability for adoration and sympathy in the entirety of their structures. It is some of the time portrayed as an extension between the psyche, body, and soul.

At the point when your Heart Chakra is all around adjusted, you will have the option to offer compassion to other people, be genuinely open, and appreciate a profound feeling of inward harmony. You may feel your feelings completely, but then additionally comprehend them on an intellectual level. Anything contrarily identified with affection can inconvenience the Heart Chakra; a separation, a melancholy procedure, a troublesome companionship, or even only an occasion of easy-going mercilessness.

- Physical Location: Directly over the heart.
- Color: Green.
- Element: Air.
- Emotional Issues and Behaviors of Blocked Heart Chakra: When the Heart Chakra is

blocked or skewed, you'll battle to identify with other individuals. You might be less empathetic than expected and might be restless. You'll ordinarily think that its harder than expected to trust, and you won't feel settled. Or maybe, you'll feel eager and displeased. A blocked Heart Chakra can likewise show physically. Some Chakra specialists figure such a misalignment might be connected to issues like hypertension and low insusceptible framework work.

## 5. The Throat Chakra (Vishuddha)

The Throat Chakra controls your self-articulation in all detects, affecting how legitimately you pass on your most profound self to the world. Your certainty, enthusiastic genuineness, and responsibility for necessities interface with this zone.

At the point when your Throat Chakra has adjusted appropriately, you will feel ready to state what you mean, be surely known by others, and talk reality in manners that are proper. As such, you'll be candid without being obtuse. Troublesome encounters with correspondence can move the Throat Chakra. For instance, an intense prospective employee meet-up or a terrible contention can move your Throat Chakra.

- Physical Location: In the throat.
- Color: Blue.
- Element: Ether.
- Emotional Issues and Behaviors of Blocked Crown Chakra: If your Crown Chakra winds up exasperates, you probably won't see much excellence on the planet by any means. You may likewise feel otherworldliness hapless and experience indications of misery. In case you're just beginning to build up this sort of square, you may very well see a decrease in general fervor or inspiration. Physically, a blocked Crown Chakra can likewise happen simultaneously as issues with physical coordination or incessant migraines.

## 6. The Third Eye Chakra (Ajna)

The Third Eye Chakra is a ground-breaking vitality source when it is functioning admirably. It decides your instinct, your arrangement with the Universe, and your capacity to see the master plan throughout everyday life.

When you have an open Third Eye chakra, you are skilled at getting signs. Trust in your premonitions and plan as per your most noteworthy objectives. Law of Attraction victories and appearance encounters identify with this sort of receptiveness. Nonetheless, the Third Eye can be skewed on the off chance that somebody is making you question your more extensive reason. Or on the other hand, in the event that you will in general prize sanity over instinct.

- Physical Location: In the focal point of your temples.
- Color: Indigo.
- Element: Extra-Sensory Perception.
- Emotional Issues and Behaviors of Blocked Third Eye Chakra: You may battle to have confidence in your more extensive reason if your Third Eye Chakra winds up blocked. In this way, you may feel there's no good reason for what you're doing, or feel it is

unimportant. You may likewise be struck by your powerlessness to decide. A few people portray this as a sentiment of mental loss of motion. On the off chance that you have a blocked Third Eye Chakra, you may experience difficulty resting, feel cumbersome, and battle to adapt new things.

## 7. The Crown Chakra (Sahasrara)

At last, the Crown Chakra, the most noteworthy chakra, is the thing that decides your otherworldly network. This chakra is in some cases called "thousand petal lotus" chakra. Given its place as the most elevated chakra, it is indispensable in making an actual existence you cherish, and in achieving a sentiment of harmony. In any case, working with it is a famously inconspicuous procedure.

At the point when everything is great, you will be tuned in to magnificence in your general surroundings. Besides, you can encounter sentiments of significant satisfaction. Life may feel beneficial, wonderful and rich. Tragically, a horrendous beneficial encounter can move the

Crown Chakra out of positive. This would then be able to make you question yourself and reason.

- Physical Location: The highest point of the head.
- Color: Violet.
- Element: Thought.
- Emotional Issues and Behaviors of Blocked Crown Chakra: If your Crown Chakra ends up aggravated, you probably won't see much excellence on the planet by any means. You may likewise feel otherworldliness afloat and experience side effects of discouragement. In case you're just beginning to build up this kind of square, you may very well see a decrease in general fervor or inspiration. Physically, a blocked Crown Chakra can likewise happen simultaneously as issues with physical coordination or constant cerebral pains.

## The Most Effective Method to Unblock Chakras

Figuring out how to unblock chakras starts with realizing why they may get blocked. A square in any of the seven chakras can show in physical disease related to that zone. It is commonly connected with some sort of close to home or mental trouble.

For instance, when your sacral chakra (beneath the midsection catch) is hindered, this can show in changes to craving and stomach related distress. Since this chakra is identified with your center character and inventiveness, the most widely recognized reasons for blockages incorporate unacceptable professions or brief period spent on self-improvement. Finding out about the hugeness and nature of each chakra will enable you to see and find blockages as they emerge.

Fortunately, it's conceivable to work out how to adjust your chakras. Correspondingly, you can expel these blockages any place they are. From contemplations that start with the one portrayed above to way of life changes and chakra yoga, there are a lot of unmistakable things you can do to move past a skewed chakra.

## Guided Chakra Meditation for Beginners

In case you're searching for contemplation for chakra adjusting, you can get familiar with a guided chakra reflection for tenderfoots that is simple, effective, and ground-breaking. Just pursue these means, giving in any event 30 seconds to everyone to encourage chakras mending.

Go to a quiet, calm spot. Sit for a couple of minutes peacefully, breathing profoundly. Give yourself a chance to learn about the pressure streaming of your body, and begin to see the scope of sensations you feel. A decent chakra contemplation includes every one of the seven chakras; start at the tailbone, envisioning a red light shining and turning at its middle. Feel it move in time with your breath.

Move center to the spot just underneath your navel, this time envisioning a warm, orange lighting turning and beating in time with the mood of your breath. Move to an inch or so over your navel. This is where you'll regularly feel love, nervousness, or zeal. Tune into an orange light turning there. Take care of the exceptionally focal point of your chest, envisioning a dazzling green light. On the off chance that you want to put a palm level on this zone as you inhale, do as such.

Concentrate on the empty of your throat, this time imagining a blue light turning and moving with the breath. Consider the space between your temples. This speaks to your third eye. See an indigo light here, getting progressively clear as it turns. At long last, picture a purple light radiating out from the highest point of your head, associating you to the vitality of the universe around you.

## Six Ways to Balance Your Chakras

Adjusting chakras, or figuring out how to how to unblock chakras, can be drawn closer in a broad scope of ways. We'll take a gander at probably the most regularly utilized and the most dominant. You can use them related, or you can pick a couple of that best suit your needs.

# 1. Contemplation for Chakra Healing

This contemplation starts with the necessary reflection procedure we've just investigated previously. It can further be adjusted for every one of the seven chakras. As you work through every one of the stages, see whether any territory feels awkward. You may likewise see trouble in imagining the development of any of the turning circles of light. Assuming this is the case, you've discovered a blockage. Concentrating on this region can help to rebalance it.

To start with, place a hand on the territory. Next, picture its cynicism or pressure depleting ceaselessly. Envision the universe emptying progressively brilliant light into the blocked chakra. Elective perceptions include purposely expanding the speed of the light pivot at that chakra. This may take some time and fixation if the chakra is substantially blocked. You may observe contemplations for chakra recuperating to be particularly successful in the event that you consolidate them with mantras (referenced underneath). It can likewise be useful to utilize fragrant healing oils like lavender and lemongrass.

## 2. Chakra Balancing Affirmations

Chakra confirmations or mantras are sounds that you rehash to yourself so as to strengthen a positive message about mending. Every one of the accompanyings can be over and again recited; ensure that you lengthen every vowel.

### Chakra Mantras

For tenderfoot perusers, every one of these confirmation mantras is spelled phonetically, so you realize how to articulate it:

Root Chakra: Laahm

Sacral Chakra: Vaahm

Sunlight based Plexus Chakra: Raahm

Heart Chakra: Yaahm

Throat Chakra: Haahm

Third eye Chakra: Ohmm

Crown Chakra: Contemplative quietness.

**Chakra Affirmations**

You ought to likewise feel allowed to structure your chakra adjusting attestations that incorporate words or expressions that allude to your objectives or saw blockages. These can be recounted into the mirror whenever. Here are some example confirmations to motivate you and kick you off:

"I feel my root chakra unblocking and welcoming positive change."

"My sacral chakra is recuperating, and I am making."

"Consistently, my sun based plexus chakra is becoming more splendid."

"I work to unblock my heart chakra and proceed onward from my torment."

"My throat chakra is adjusting, and my words are getting to be more clear."

"I unblock my third eye chakra, explaining my vision and my instinct."

**3. Chakra Yoga**

As investigated when we took a gander at the historical backdrop of chakras, adjusting the chakras is an antiquated practice. Therefore, yoga has for quite some time been utilized to unblock the chakras and help individuals to progress toward becoming sensitive to their vitality. Chakra yoga urges you to control, flex, and reposition portions of the body that are connected to specific chakras. Thusly, this animates them and advances the progression of positive vitality all through the whole framework. In the event that you realize some fundamental yoga positions, they are likely previously helping you to improve and keep up excellent chakra wellbeing.

For an apprentice, all that is indeed required is to rehearse nonexclusive yoga consistently. Also, remember chakra blockages and pressure discharges all through. In any case, there are additionally explicit chakra yoga methods that you can proceed to learn in the event that you need to propel your comprehension. Specifically, there are five represents that intend to focus on the first five chakras.

## 4. Change Your Diet

In the event that you've been examining how to adjust your chakras, you'll have seen that diet and way of life are said to assume an exceptional job. To adapt your chakras, distinguish which ones are blocked and after that eat a more significant amount of the accompanying nourishments and herbs relying upon which chakras you need to take a shot at:

- Root Chakra: Elderberry, strawberries, tomatoes, raspberries.
- Sacral Chakra: Parsley, oranges, chime peppers.
- Solar Plexus Chakra: Chamomile, bananas, lemons.
- Heart Chakra: Lemon medicine, green vegetables, green apples.
- Throat Chakra: Sage, blueberries, dark currants.
- Third eye Chakra: Spruce, indigo vegetables.
- Crown Chakra: Thyme, eggplant, red grapes.

In the event that you make a propensity for joining a broad scope of hues in your sustenance (for example in natural product plates of mixed greens, pasta, and soups), you can work to adjust the majority of your chakras during each dinner of the day.

## 5. Chakra Healing Reiki

Reiki includes setting your hands on better places on the body so as to encourage positive vitality move, negative vitality evacuation, and by and large recuperating. Chakra mending reiki places utilizing this system on the particular territories where each chakra is found. You can either hold your palm over the territory or spot it level on the skin.

On the off chance that you know which specific chakra or chakras are blocked, concentrate the chakra recuperating reiki process on that spot. Notwithstanding, in the event that you need to advance by and considerable prosperity and joy (or feel a blockage yet don't know where it's found), specialists suggest that you work through each of the chakras thus.

In time, individuals who practice chakra mending reiki may figure out how to "sense" blockages in themselves as well as other people, just by gradually passing their hand along the body and seeing zones that vibe lopsided. Notwithstanding, even amateurs can see enormous advantages from the fundamental advances sketched out above.

## 6. EFT for Chakras

At last, EFT, the passionate opportunity strategy, can likewise be utilized to adjust the seven chakras. EFT has demonstrated incredibly compelling for individuals who battle with traditional types of treatment. Also, it very well may be managed with no extraordinary mastery or gear.

In a word, EFT (which is once in a while just called "tapping") includes delicately contacting zones on the body that are associated with vitality focuses. While you tap your fingers on the fitting vitality focus, you center around the issue you're encountering, and on the objective, you have at the top of the priority list.

EFT for chakras is sensibly precise and instinctive. For instance, on the off chance that you have done a chakra contemplation and understood that there is a blockage in your third eye chakra, tapping on the territory between your foreheads can discharge pressure and advance viable vitality stream. As you do as such, envision the shining vitality focus becoming more splendid and moving quicker, similarly as you do during your chakra reflection method.

# CHAPTER TWO

## THE THREE PILLARS OF REIKI

Other than the five REIKI standards, Dr. Usui showed his REIKI framework, which depends on these columns: GASSHO, REIJI-HO, and CHIRYO.

**GASSHO**

GASSHO truly signifies "two hands meeting up," and Dr. Usui showed a contemplation by the name of GASSHO MEDITATION. This contemplation was drilled each time toward the start of his REIKI workshops/gatherings. It is intended to be rehearsed for 20-30 minutes in the wake of getting up as well as in the prior night resting. Gassho should be possible alone or in a gathering. Gathering reflections are a superb encounter since the vitality increments along ways past the aggregate of the individual member's energies.

Gassho Meditation is easy to such an extent that people of all ages can do it. Following three days of training, you will know based on sentiments, whether it is "ideal" for you. At that point, if conceivable, you should rehearse it consistently for at any rate three months. In any case, if following a couple of days, you have a sentiment of anxiety, touchiness, or some other type of disturbance, this intercession may potentially not be reasonable for you. Few out of every odd prescription works for every patient. At that point, you can essentially attempt it again following half a month.

- When doing Gassho, plunk down with shut eyes and hands put together with before your heart chakra. Center your whole consideration at the point where the two center fingers meet.
- If it is excruciating for you to hold your hands collapsed together along these lines for twenty minutes or somewhere in the vicinity, at that point let your hands (keeping them together) gradually sink down to your lap

into an agreeable position and keep on thinking.

- Energy wonders may likewise happen, for example, your hands or spine ending up exceptionally warm: watch this however don't give yourself a chance to be affected by it. Continuously return your concentration to the point where your two center fingers meet.

- If you should change your sitting position, at that point, move in moderate movement: intentionally and deliberately. It is simpler to think when the spinal section is as straight as could be expected under the circumstances, and the head doesn't tilt either advance, in reverse or to the side. Envision that your head is appended to an inflatable loaded up with helium, which delicately keeps it in the ideal position. On the off chance that you have back issues or are not used to sitting, you can sit on a seat with a back, with a pad or pad behind you, or with your back inclined toward a divider. There are fundamentally no issues with reflection while resting, and then again, actually it welcomes us to nod off!

## REIJI-HO

Converted into English, REIJI signifies "sign of the REIKI power," and HO signifies "techniques" (In Hawayo Takata's diary, this strategy was referenced in a section of May 1936). REIJI-HO comprises of three short ceremonies that are completed before every treatment: -

**Fold your hands before your heart chakra in the Gassho act.**

What's more, close your eyes. Presently associate with the REIKI control. This is exceptionally basic: Ask the REIKI capacity to move through you. Inside a couple of moments, you will see how it streams. Maybe you will feel it enter through your crown chakra or you may see it first in your heart chakra or in your grasp (it doesn't make a difference wherein part of your body the sign initially happens). You can likewise utilize the separation (Hon Sha Ze Sho Nen) Symbol to interface with the REIKI control. Rehash the desire multiple times in your mind that REIKI may stream, at that point send the Mental/Emotional (Sei He Ki) Symbol and seal everything with the Power (Cho Ku Rei) Symbol. When you feel the vitality, proceed to the subsequent stage.

**Pray for the recuperation and additionally soundness of the patient/customer on all levels.**

Here recall that we don't have a clue what is "great" or "awful" for our patients/customers, why they "need" or have a specific ailment thus, put the expressions "recuperation" and "wellbeing" in the hands of the REIKI control and become a channel for it (devoting it, obviously, for their most noteworthy great) – they will get whatever is directly for them.

**Now hold your collapsed delivers front of your third eye and request.**

REIKI has the capacity to control your hands to where the vitality is required. From the start, this method may appear to be unusual to you, negating what you have officially found out about REIKI. Be that as it may, your hands recognize what's going on, so figure out how to confide in them. We are generally essentially instinctive – we simply need to figure out how to tune in to the motivation that is as of now there and "decipher" it effectively. How you connect with your instinct and in what region it shows itself is diverse for every person.

Ultimately, the third mainstay of reiki is chiryo, the treatment. This is the place you give the reiki to your customer. There are uniform treatment focuses, and ones through experimentation and training that you find without anyone else. The session is generally exceptionally unwinding for the customer, and both the specialist and customer can get direction and recuperating from the treatment.

This is an exceptionally basic clarification of what every column involves in the three mainstays of reiki custom. Custom is the thing that interfaces us together to express our goals. We are such phenomenal vitality sources. With the correct recipe, a seed of goal alongside assertions and an association, your aim is made, and your association is developed. With training, direction, and practice, these means will help you in developing your association with yourself and the reiki source.

# CHAPTER THREE

## BIOENERGETICS THEORY

There is no settled upon hypothesis for how Reiki may function, and its component of activity is as yet obscure. Therefore, Reiki is liable to the analysis levelled at other CAM modalities by cynics: it can't be strong in light of the fact that it comes up short on a known natural system of activity. As David Hufford has contended, verifiable in this view is the conviction that CAM cases will be demonstrated to be 'genuine' or 'false' based on present logical information, furthermore, that "the acknowledgment of any hypothetically unrealistic cases would require the deserting of current logical learning." This obviously closes all request before it starts, ruling out making associations between hypotheses hidden energy recuperating practices, for example, Reiki, Therapeutic touch, or Qi gong, and those rising in different parts of the ordinary sciences.

The ideas fundamental energy treatments, for example, Reiki have hypothetical shared traits with an assortment of models in material science, none of which have been tentatively connected with drug or clinical results. Models in bioelectromagnetism, quantum material science, and superstring theory18 are reliable with Asian Sacred writing in recommending that inconspicuous vibration might be the substratum of reality as we probably are aware of it, and hence such vibration may have a task to carry out in wellbeing and ailment. For instance, Jan Walleczek24 and Abe Liboff25 in the field of bioelectromagnetism offer valid logical help for the potential job of the powers of inconspicuous bioelectromagnetic fields in physiological procedures. Walleczek specifically has convincingly exhibited that inconspicuous attractive fields can have quantifiable communications with organic frameworks in the region of redox potential and hydroxylation responses. In spite of the fact that this zone of research is in its beginning times, these associations recommend that the hypothetical underpinnings of Reiki and other energy treatments may not be in direct inconsistency to logical models.

Reiki vibration is comprehended to be drawn through the professional as per the beneficiary's need, inside the capacity of the specialist to convey the vibration. Starting understudies regularly think that it's hard to get a handle on that non-doing can be so powerful. The progression of Reiki is accepted to increment as the expert turns out to be deep down progressively. Still, an understanding obtained uniquely through star ached practice. The way that the vibrational stream is drawn by the beneficiary takes into consideration extraordinary adaptability and simplicity of conveyance. While an expert's capacity to be a channel for the vibrations may differ, there is, at last, no off-base method. Reiki's self-administrative system blocks "overdosing" — even a dry wipe just retains to immersion. Experienced specialists guarantee to see when the mending vibrational stream diminishes, at which time they move to the following hand position. Beneficiaries regularly sense a vibrational stream, now and again feeling warmth or coolness, or floods of unwinding all through their body, or in explicit zones that could possibly relate to where the expert's hands are put. Such encounters might be proof of an unobtrusive entrainment impact, like that of sound mending, whereby Reiki vibrations adjust the beneficiary's biofield to more prominent concordance. Reiki is accepted to rebalance the biofield, along these lines reinforcing the body's capacity to mend and expanding foundational protection from stress. It seems to diminish pressure and invigorate self-mending by unwinding and maybe by resetting the resting tone of the autonomic sensory system. Defenders of Reiki accept this may prompt upgrade of insusceptible framework work and expanded endorphin creation.

**Bioenergy Laws**

Bioenergy laws are a definitive zenith of my examination on how the atmosphere and bodywork, just as on the instrument of rising and vanishing of an ailment. They demonstrate that every one of the illnesses, mental and natural, showed up because of the breakdown of the vitality structure of the quality. An infection cannot rise if everything is OK with the suitable fragment of the atmosphere and, the other way around, one can't discuss wellbeing if the air is harmed.

So as to orchestrate the vitality structure of the quality and body with the four bioenergy laws, the dark and the white bioenergy, just as their common proportion inside the air must be advanced; the vitality stabilizer, which speaks to the core of the air, needs to work typically; the white bioenergy in every one of the purposes of the atmosphere must have a similar worth, for example, it must be homogeneously conveyed; and that the recurrence of vitality is as per the one is given to human-animal categories.

**Bioenergetics Therapy**

Bioenergetics, created by Dr. Alexander Lowen, is a progressive treatment that uses the language of the body to mend the issues of the brain. This treatment joins physical agony, muscle strain, and postural issue with perspectives, exhibiting that stifled feelings, despondency, and outrage can square vitality stream and cause physical trouble. An individual is an incredible entirety experience, every one of which is enlisted as a part of his character and organized in his body. Feelings are, in essence, occasions; truly developments or movement inside the body that by and large bring about some outward activity.

## Develop AURA

The use of bioenergy laws by wearing a charm or through my mending treatment guarantees the ideal working of the atmosphere and prompts significant changes in its appearance. On the off chance that we contrast it with the ordinary one, which is portrayed by red tones, this develops quality comprises of two essential hues: brilliant yellow and dull blue. The focal point of the yellow vitality center is really of the shade of old gold and is arranged inside the mid-region and chest. Waves start throbbing, similar to heart thumps, from the yellow vitality center, and go to the part of the arrangement filling it with liberal vitality.

## Avoidance

The lifestyle and thinking about the cutting edge man prompts ordinary pressure and negative musings, the consequences of which are constant natural and dysfunctional behaviors. Their overwhelming impacts spread further and make the narrow mindedness of various types that toxic substance relational connections inside the family and companions, and are one of the primary drivers of wars. Does it need to be like this? Is there a fix to this wickedness?

The fix can be found in an efficient counteractive action program that would change the manner in which individuals think and would prompt maintaining a strategic distance from upsetting circumstances. Notwithstanding, we as a whole need to change independently. Is it difficult to blend one's desires with one's capacities, rather than attempting to do it the other route round? The person who is malcontented with their activity should attempt to secure the position that suits the person in question better, supposing that one is sick, one isn't prepared to do any activity. Is it difficult to endure individuals around you? Would we be able to live regardless of whether we are not the ones in power? Can we, in certain circumstances, base our activities on reason, rather than only on our souls. Would it be advisable for us to pursue this, our wellbeing would be better and progressively balanced out?

## Recuperating Sources Other Than Human

I have prevailed with regards to initiating every one of the energies that a human body can discharge for mending purposes, yet I have still not been completely satisfied with the accomplished impacts. What can anyone do? Proceeding with my exploration, in the next months, I vanquished another territory – mending energies, the wellsprings of which are not inside people. I was step by step enabled to enact and coordinate countless energies towards a patient. Their sources can be isolated into three huge gatherings: fake ones, common ones, and otherworldly ones.

**Counterfeit sources are:**

- Pyramids, which gather the recuperating energy from the space around them, in light of their shape. The vitality at that point streams along the pyramid's edges towards its top. When I request this, energies of the four pyramids close to Cairo are assembled into a little cloud, which is promptly moved over the patient, and he gets it through a bar.

- Old houses of worship, where the mending energy is produced along the vertical edges of dividers up to the top, and from that point it very well may be coordinated through a bar towards the patient.

The force and nature of the recuperating energy from the man-developed sources rely upon the size of the structure, its shape, age, and the motivation behind those structures.

**Regular sources include:**

- Gravitational recuperating vitality of the Earth and other heavenly bodies the mending vitality of which can raise a patient's invulnerable level;

- Healing segment of energies of every heavenly body, which is experienced immediately, and utilized in basic states, particularly against torment;

- Cosmic vitality, whose recuperating part speaks to the most dominant wellspring of dim bioenergy known to man. After I ask in this way, it originates from all bearings and packs into a little cloud, and sends a bar to the patient, until it is spent.

These energies are distinctive from various perspectives, yet their common point is that the recuperating vitality is similar dim bioenergy radiated from hands and chakras, and the one with constrained limits.

Nonetheless, the most significant gathering of recuperating vitality sources are profound sources, and they are the iridescent body, Energy Cloud, Christ's Energy, and God's Energy. The power that empowers me to send an intrigue to recuperate brought a great deal of fervor and delight to me. On the off chance that I set aside feelings and otherworldly angles and watch just the mending vitality that these creatures direct towards patients, I reach the resolution this is about an incredibly smart vitality. At the point when this vitality is actuated after my intrigue, and it goes to the patient, it initially investigates the wellbeing of his atmosphere and body to the most modest subtleties. At that point, it intercedes with its mending power any place it is important, for the most part inside the quality. Should it not have a reasonable kind of vitality, it here and there draws in it from some other source and carries it to the patient. It, along these lines, does basically everything, without my or any other person's cooperation, obviously, just on the off chance that I ask it to. Other than mending, these profound creatures are prepared to support me, after I ask them to, in some different everyday issues.

This part in the field of research has to lead me to the way that every one of the diseases happens because of the lopsidedness in the vitality structure inside the air, and furthermore that the ailments vanish once the air is brought to its ideal state. There is a more all-inclusive route than treating specific ailments. By orchestrating the emanation, one influences every one of the sicknesses, natural and mental, the ones the patient thinks about, and those, which have not yet shown up. It likewise anticipates the event of new ceaseless illnesses.

# Seeing Bioenergy

Bioenergy can't be enlisted with our faculties. Be that as it may, there are individuals who have the extra tactile recognition and can see different paranormal wonders, including bioenergy. An additional sense saw the dim bioenergy as a dainty dark white fog, which is surrounding us, and which comprises of exceptionally little white spots. One of the most intriguing marvels is seeing the atmosphere. Utilizing the radiesthesia technique, I understood that the air has ten layers of various hues, measurements, and bioenergy thickness. The extra sense saw these layers in various hues and their best subtleties. As indicated by him, a solid atmosphere has the main layer, which envelopes the body, and it is the shade of light, while the subsequent one is straightforward. Layers that pursue are: whitish, dull red, splendid red, red mists, little pink mists, foggy, white, and brilliant white bars.

While concentrating principle chakras, the extra sense saw that they all appeared to be unique. Toward the part of the bargaining channel, the additional sense saw the organ of extrasensory recognition - the third eye, which stays undeveloped until actuated. The third eye looks like a breezy student made of sensory tissue. While mending with chakras, a slight brilliant pillar rises up out of the bio-healer's third eye. I considered this pillar a pilot bar. It goes vertically upwards, and after that on a level plane right to the patient any place he might be, and brings down itself straightforwardly onto him, that is, his influenced organ. Essentially at a similar minute an exceptionally solid vitality bar, very like a spotlight pillar, rises up out of the utilized chakra and arrives at the patient after the roughly parallel way to that of the pilot light. The more grounded shaft promptly begins to fill the influenced organ with dim bioenergy, which could be found in the difference in shading from dim dark to light dim, practically white. After the filling procedure is finished, the two shafts are put out, and the recuperating is finished.

The whole procedure is sorted out by the glowing body, through its directions given to the third eye. If there should be an occurrence of the concurrent radiation of at least three chakras, bars don't experience individual chakras, yet are altogether coordinated towards the focal channel, and in the wake of entering it, they rise through the seventh chakra as one in number shaft.

## The Sensation of Bioenergy Healing

Two individuals partake in the bioenergy mending or move bio-healer and his patient. The mode and power of every one of them experience the session is unique. The healer feels gentle prickles on palms or fingers, sticks, and needles in their grasp, or an unpretentious current of air, warmth on their palms, and frequently they don't feel anything. While recuperating with chakras, paying little respect to their more grounded intensity of radiation, the bio-healer feels only a mellow sensation. The patient regularly encounters warmth, needles, and sticks, gooseflesh, air current, once in a while chills, unsteadiness, weight at the back of his head, a suspending sensation, a sensation as though one is riding on little waves, gentle agonies as well. There are patients who feel nothing; however, that doesn't defame the constructive outcomes of recuperating.

# Negative Thoughts and Stress as Main Causes of Illnesses

Individuals have for since quite a while ago accepted that pressure, negative contemplations, and feelings could prompt natural and mental sicknesses. As of late, present-day prescription likewise concedes that pressure certainly affects the development of sicknesses. My exploration work in the field of paranormal has demonstrated that, in the event that we set aside wounds and hurtful radiation, at that point pressure, negative musings and feelings speak to the fundamental driver of over 80% ailments. Negative contemplations are discontent with oneself and one's work, contempt, begrudge, control battle, dread, pity, and grieving. Our negative idea is a vitality wave, which is discharged from the mind and instigates harm on the vitality structure of the air and body. The degree of the harm relies upon the force, sort, and span of negative musings and stress. The results of these harms are constant sicknesses, both natural and mental. Regardless of whether the sickness is irresistible, the above may prompt the colossal advancement of infections and microscopic organisms.

Stress and contrary contemplations are the reason for the greatest wickedness that influences mankind and leads not exclusively to intense and incessant sicknesses, yet additionally makes terrible relations among individuals, absence of resilience of different types, religious, national and racial. It is one of the primary drivers of wars. That is the reason it is essential to sort out a counteractive action from this fiendishness. This anticipation should prompt the manner in which people think and to the most extreme evading of distressing circumstances.

## Effect of Stress and Negative Thoughts on White Bioenergy

The flood of the negative considerations vitality and the pressure vitality field can't kill, can't devastate the white bioenergy. Be that as it may, if the dim bioenergy is pulverized, concordance between the dark and white bioenergy is annihilated, in light of the fact that the white bioenergy overpowers, and this prompts the crumbling of the express the quality is in. Also, since the jam entered the meridians, the progression of white bioenergy is backed off, or ended. That is the reason the measure of the white bioenergy on its way towards the vitality stabilizer is diminished; its working ends up more fragile, and it scatters a little measure of white bioenergy. As an outcome, we have the white bioenergy heaped up in one piece of the air, and less white bioenergy in the other. This is the best approach to significantly obliterate the air's agreement that was there before the unsafe musings happened.

# CHAPTER FOUR

## THE WAYS OF DEALING WITH NEGATIVE ENERGIES

Do you here and there feel like your body has a "completion" to it, that you are holding a lot of things in your body, it feels awkward, strange and you can't clarify what it is? You could be holding a lot of energy in your body, and I'm not discussing positive, cheerful life; however, the thoughtful which leaves you feeling depleted, on edge and tired. You may feel total overpower and your body goes into survival mode as you attempt and understand what is new with you. You feel extraordinary, such as everything is excessively troublesome or easily overlooked details feel like serious issues.

This happens to a more significant number of individuals than you can envision – particularly sensitives and empaths, because of your interesting fiery makeup, your vigorous limits are slim and open, which can prompt you taking on different people groups feelings. Negative energy could likewise be connected to items like legacies or can be felt more in one room of a house than another. Now and again, negative energy could also be brought about by otherworldly existences. If so, you can find a way to clear your items and home by utilizing some of what I propose in my tips underneath. You can likewise request that a Healer help you clear negative vitality from your home.

To have the option to draw on your qualities as an empath or delicate realize that you can figure out how to secure and clear yourself. Your life needs uncommon consideration, and when you figure out how to fortify and wash down your energy, you will be in a superior position to manage negative vitality and by and large feel much improved and have more life yourself.

Your vitality framework comprises of your energy body which is called your "Emanation" and the principle energy focuses which are designated "Chakras." Your air is egg molded around your body and secures your vitality field by making an enthusiastic "shield" among you and other individuals' energy. In the event that it is energetic, beautiful, and reliable, you will feel empowered and prepared to take on anything which comes to your direction.

The fiery focuses in your body give life power vitality to the encompassing organs and keep you sound and stable on the off chance that they are clear and without vigorous squares. On the off chance that you are effectively enthusiastically overpowered, you may have an irregularity in your chakras – for the most part in the root chakra, which is situated toward the part of the arrangement and which associates you to the Earth. In the event that this chakra is vigorously powerless, you regularly feel ungrounded, once in a while even "scattered" and this can lead effectively to fiery overpower by not occupying your body wholly.

Fortunately, with a couple of basic purging strategies, you can figure out how to effortlessly fortify and secure your vitality field, making you stronger to other individuals' energies. You will turn out to be vigorously more grounded and will have more vitality to create a fantastic most and do the things you cherish. I'm natural and have consistently been profoundly delicate to individuals' feelings. Before I realized how to secure and clear myself, I used to stroll around like a wipe truly sucking up individuals' energy like water, which left me feeling like a unique individual generally days. In the course of the most recent year, mainly doing vitality function as a Reiki Healer, I needed to figure out how to clear my vitality all the time. I've genuinely realized what functions admirably for me and its presently part of my day by day/week after week schedule.

**ONE: Spend Time in Nature**

There is nothing superior to natural air, daylight, and the ocean to gather up negative vitality. Surrounding you, and all through the whole universe, circles life energy. It exists not just as a vitality field around each living thing, yet besides flows through the Earth, through the environment around us and all through nature.

The progression of this vitality interfaces everything that exists, and you, as a living being, are taking in this vitality at each minute. You are continually drawing this life vitality into your vitality field, and it is this vitality that supports your life. When you imagine nature's energy to encompass you, you direct the spirit with an easy goal to enable you to clear and recuperate your vitality.

Wind and Sun – Stand outside and feel the breeze and sun all over. Feel the intensity of the breeze which encompasses you and imagines sending all negative vitality in your body to be diverted with the breeze. Feel the glow of the sun all over and believe it was stimulating every cell in your body.

The Ocean – The ocean is an incredible vitality chemical, and the salt from the ocean has a remarkable capacity to retain negative vitality. Take a dip in the sea or remain with your feet in the waves and envision it washing endlessly any negative energy. Envision the negative energy venturing out onto the ocean and leaving you unadulterated and scrubbed indeed.

Walk Barefoot in Nature – The root chakra which is situated toward the part of the bargain and associates you into the Earth gives you a sentiment of security and insurance when it's enthusiastically solid. The snappiest and most effortless approach to fortify it is to remove your shoes and walk shoeless on the Earth. By interfacing with the Earth and envisioning your "foundations" associating with the focal point of the Earth, it encourages you to feel grounded and ready to fend off negative energies.

## TWO: Using Your Breath

Profound breathing causes you to let go of remaining vitality held inside your body. Start by making deep, careful breaths and feel how your breath moves the energy around your body. Envision taking in a real-life and breathing out any negative life. Breathing is a piece of the existing power which invigorates our body and encourages oxygen stream to our organs to keep them stable.

Have you at any point wanted to yawn? Take the plunge! I frequently stretch during a Reiki session or after a Reiki session, not because I'm exhausted however I'm discharging vitality. Yawning is the body's normal response to giving up – it additionally causes us to carry more oxygen into the blood and move more carbon dioxide out of the blood.

## THREE: Dance to Call in Your Joy

Put on your main tune and shake your body like nobody's viewing. I adore moving and singing as it enables discharge to feel high endorphins which makes me feel positive and inspired by and by. While moving envisions, shaking off any negative vitality and explores positive, upbeat vitality flood your body.

Music invigorates the cerebrum's reward focuses, while move animates the arrival of endorphins and gives us a characteristic high, notwithstanding expanding our digestion and bloodstream, so it's incredible exercise as well. Moving carries happiness to you and sends positive vibrations out to the universe, and it likewise raises your vitality vibration. When you move, you feel an "aliveness" in your spirit, and when you are in this condition of bliss, you can draw in an unfaltering truth of energy.

## FOUR: Use Sound to Dispel Negative Energy

Sound is transformational and recuperating on such a significant number of levels. I have a Shanti Bowl, which I use during reflection. I adore it as it produces delightful consonant music which summons a profound reflective and serene state. These "singing" bowls help balance the body's chakras, wipe out pressure, and advance comprehensive recuperating.

You can likewise tune in to music which refines and wash down your vitality – playing high vibration music can help dissipate negative energy and get change our vitality bodies and around our home.

## FIVE: Bring Light into Your Life

I cherish utilizing candles, they smell dazzling and make a warm, relieving the feeling. You can likewise use candles to clear your energy. Light a white flame and set your aim to ensure and clear your vitality by saying "I devote this flame to the light and request insurance to encompass me" – envision the light of the candle encompassing you and enable your Angels and Guides to surround you with assurance. You will probably consume with extreme heat any negative vitality. Seeing it, announce your aim to have all negative life enter the fire. On a bit of paper, compose words for clearing negative energies. Something like "I currently discharge, copy and clear everything negative influencing my wellbeing…. my life…. my vitality". Ensure you discard the bit of paper – the demonstration of dropping it implies you are relinquishing the negative energy.

## SIX: Use Essential Oils and Incense

I adore utilizing incense around my home anyway a few people think that it's hard to endure the smell of smear sticks or fragrance so diffusing necessary oils and making a "smirch mix" could be an incredible option. I've come to love utilizing essential oils and use them around my home to wash down, inspire, quiet, and mend my home and my family. Here is a portion of my preferred oils to help clear and inspire – you can snatch yours here.

Most basic oils will affect our feelings. They are breathed in and rapidly go through our nasal entries to the smell tactile gathering nerves.

Basic Oil    Used For

Lavender     Clears out energies that won't leave a space.

White Sage     Neutralizes current pessimism and makes a clairvoyant shield against strains.

Juniper     Is clearing and attracts positive, defensive vitality and advances detoxification.

Myrrh     Transforms harmful condition, joined with different oils it builds their power

Neroli     Helps with tension and frenzy.

Bergamot     Releases passionate torment is a fantastic upper and assuages pressure

Frankincense     Used principally for purging and sanitization.

## SEVEN: Crystals for Positive Energy Flow

I've lost check of what number of precious stones I have in my home. I completely adore them and use them routinely to support my vitality. All precious stones have their remarkable properties to help lift or bright energy from multiple points of view.

I particularly love amethyst, it's beautiful and secures me against negative vitality and mystic assaults. Obsidian is an exceptionally incredible precious stone – it will try to clean negative energy in its region, additionally inside the air, making this a helpful stone. Continuously wash down your precious stones all the time to dispose of any negative vitality ingested.

**EIGHT: Himalayan Salt Lamps and Salt Baths**

Himalayan Salt is the most valuable, cleanest salt on earth. It was shaped around 250 million years prior and started from when the universe was utterly immaculate and with no ecological effect. It retains water and particles from the air and takes on positive particles with them. At that point, when the warmed salt discharges scrubbed water vapour over into the air, it removes harmful particles. As a precious artificial stone for both clairvoyant insurance and purging dull vitality, Pink Himalayan Salt is a moderate and straightforward to-utilize answer for disposing of substantial energy that is overloading you.

It is additionally known to sanitize, purge, and freshen up the air, builds vitality levels, decreases sensitivity and asthma, lessens pressure; however, above all, it kills electromagnetic radiation from electronic gadgets. There is nothing superior to having a long absorb the shower following a furious day. In the event that you don't have Himalayan Salt Bath Crystals, utilize unadulterated ocean salt, and incorporate a loosening up salt shower. Salt will cleanse you and expel negative energies from your body.

Here is my extraordinary shower douse to help discharge negative vitality:

- Add to running warm water in your rain.
- 1 to 2 cups of Himalayan salt precious stones or Sea Salt. Guarantee the salt completely breaks down before getting into the water.
- 2 to 3 drops every one of frankincense, geranium, lavender, and sandalwood.
- Soak for at any rate 20 minutes on the off chance that you can. Appreciate!

## NINE: Waterfall Energy

Probably the snappiest ways I purify my vitality is to utilize "cascade vitality." Necessarily picture remaining under a cascade and feel the water purge any negative energy. I likewise "paint" my principle access to my home with cascade vitality to guarantee any individual who strolls into my house is "washed clean."

## TEN: Smudging with Sage

White Sage has been utilized for refinement and purifying for quite a long time. Smirching your consecrated space, your home or office, or even your body with sage resembles washing up or doing a profound supernatural purging.

Instructions to Protect Yourself

- Imagine a Protective Shield Around You
- Do this representation when you work with or are around individuals always, you are going to go into an especially upsetting circumstance or basically to expand your

vigorous and enthusiastic strength after some time.

- Close your eyes
- Try and feel or sense your atmosphere (it may be challenging to do to start with; however, after a little practice, it will wind up simpler).
- Try and sense where your fiery limits end. Your air could be open very wide or a lot nearer to your body.
- Imagine extending your vigorous limits outward a couple of centimetres around your body.
- When you feel or sense it, picture the vitality around your body as a thick section of splendid white light or the shading blue or purple as a resistive divider or shield. I discover purple works truly well for me.
- Go with your impulses and pick what feels directly for you.
- After a touch of training, you ought to have the option to promptly envision the shading around you so you can rapidly ensure your vitality field.

- Finish off by asking your Guides, Angels, and the universe to encompass you with security now and consistently.

# CHAPTER FIVE

## Step by Step Guidance On Hand Position for Reiki Healing Techniques

As indicated by Reiki lessons, the Reiki energy is keen for it realizes where to go and what to do. The Reiki professional is told to enable the energy to stream, without coordinating the energy. It isn't essential to consider arcane speculations of the universe so as to utilize Reiki. The straightforward goal makes the Reiki vitality stream, and the purpose coordinates the vitality. The best thing for the specialist to do is nothing, however, to escape the way and enable the energy to do its work. In Reiki, there are mostly conventional and crucial hand positions instructed in Reiki accreditation courses that are utilized to advance energy equalization and help with mending to different zones of the body. Contingent upon your specific medical problem, additional time might be spent on one zone than another during a Reiki treatment. This chapter features the original Reiki hand positions, as a rule. A portion of the hand positions might be discarded as well as they may happen in an alternate request during a session. Minor departure from these positions may likewise be made, contingent upon your individual needs. In case you're going in for your first treatment, these are the positions you can by and large hope to be utilized, as they are reasonable to most treatment sessions. Each situation is intended to adjust the energies here and evacuates stuck energies there with the goal that you can start to unwind, decrease pressure and enable space for your body to rest and mend and to work all the more ideally. On the off chance that you need specific consideration set on one region, do tell your professional. Ordinarily, your specialist will have the option to detect territories inside the hand places that need additional attention you might not have even known required it.

**What's in Store During a Reiki Treatment**

During a Reiki session, a customer lays smoothly on a back rub table or is at times situated on a seat. There is no control of tissue as in back rub or bodywork that happens, yet only an exceptionally delicate hand weight. Also, not at all like back rub treatment, you are in every case entirely dressed during a Reiki session. The session is generally done peacefully with insignificant talking, except if obviously, you wish to convey something to your specialist; at that point, it is significant that you do so expeditiously during the session. Your Reiki professional may play calm, alleviating mood melodies or nature sounds. On the off chance that you are awkward or could be increasingly agreeable, for instance, if the music is diverting or in the event that you want to avoid a specific Reiki hand position, let your specialist know previously or during your session.

**The Reiki "Contact"**

Reiki is performed with either delicate, static weight from the specialist's hands on customary hand position territories, or with their hands drifting a couple of crawls over your body. Reiki works similarly also in either case so in the event that you want not to be contacted legitimately with any of the majority of the hand positions and favour the drifting technique if it's not too much trouble impart that to your expert previously or during your session. Touchy or isolated regions are never contacted during a Reiki session. Regardless of whether you have a medical problem in a touchy or private zone, it is against a Reiki Professional Practitioner's Code of Ethics to physically contact individual or delicate zones. Your Reiki Practitioner needs you to have the most unwinding and pleasant experience as could be expected under the circumstances while you appreciate this immortal technique for Japanese vitality work for pressure decrease, unwinding, and health.

## Reiki treatment convention

There is a treatment convention generally educated to Reiki specialists which includes a progression of hand positions. These positions are very much separated along the customer's body, and together they give great inclusion of the customer's whole body. While the vitality goes where it is most required, it is frequently watched the vibrancy remains close to where the professional has set their hands. By covering all pieces of the body equally, the patient will, as a matter of course, get the ideal treatment.

These hand positions act like "preparing wheels" for professionals to start rehearsing Reiki. With experience, the person should don't hesitate to test dependent on the requirements existing apart from everything else. The photos which pursue originate from the book Essential Reiki: A Complete Guide to an Ancient Healing Art (the book offers authorization to recreate the images for educating materials). Notwithstanding the positions appeared for the front of the body, there is a coordinating arrangement of positions for the back. Behind the neck, behind the heart, behind the kidneys, and on the sacrum (tailbone).

While any arrangement of hand positions is just a rule, some Reiki Masters demand utilizing only the hand positions. Most Reiki specialists build up mechanical or different techniques lead the hands to positions to be used in each mending session. One regular strategy is the scope wherein the specialist clears their hands through the customer's vitality field searching for problem areas. These demonstrate spots requiring mending vitality.

**Body security and moral practice**

One note about body security. Commonly the professional must place their hands extremely close (or on) body parts most consider to be private (genitalia). Since Reiki treats the whole body, it's ideal to not let such body parts well enough alone for treatment. A few people need mending in their genitalia or other private body parts. Simultaneously there are matters of security to ensure, and the danger of maltreatment by the professional. Fare thee well and expertly do your work.

Every professional has their particular manner of dealing with this. It's excellent to advise the customer and ask authorization before the session so that there are no curveballs. There are a few different ways to work in these zones without straightforwardly contacting the customer's body and without trading off the mending session. First is for the customer to put their very own hands on their body; at that point, the expert places their hands over the customer's hands. The expert should "pillar" the vitality through the customer's hands. Another alternative is for the specialist to hold their hands over those regions, with no contacting, and shaft the energy from a slight separation. Ultimately the separation mending images can be utilized.

## Specialist comfort

Expert solace is very significant while rehearsing Reiki. A full treatment can without much of a stretch keep going for an hour, and if the patient is lying on the floor by what method can the professional stay agreeable slouch over for that long? Better is for the patient to be situated in a seat that gives the simple expert access to their entire body. Back rub tables are generally excellent for Reiki since they can be balanced, are agreeable, and enables the patient to loosen up more thoroughly. A few organizations make tables implied explicitly for Reiki which allows a move around the seat to go underneath the table.

**Hand positions**

Position 1

Palms of your hands are put against your face, measuring your hands over your eyes delicately and fingers upon your temple. No weight required - contact softly!

Position 2

Spot your hands on the two sides of your head, impact points of your hands resting close to your ears, fingertips contacting at the crown.

Position 3

Here the hands are supporting the head, with the fingers twisted around the occipital edge. Get into this situation by tenderly shaking the head into one side, slide the other hand under the head, shake the head into that hand, move the other hand under the head, and afterward shake the administrator, so it's focused on two sides. This is simpler shown than depicted.

Position 4

Here the hands are held over the throat and thymus. You may discover customers awkward with the hands over the highest point of the throat, as it may help them to remember stifling, and you may think that it's better to put the hands under the throat instead of above it.

Position 5

This is over the heart and heart chakra. The heart chakra is situated between the bosoms. You ought to pick your hand positions well here. Note that while Reiki gets from Qi Gong, and subsequently the "chakras" ought to be unfamiliar to Reiki, the "chakras" are part of the human vitality framework, and the Tibetans and Hindu's called them a particular something, while the Chinese considered them another.

Position 6

Hands might be put delicately on your upper guts.

Position 7

The professional may put their hands on your sunlight based plexus territory or mid-stomach area.

Position 8

The specialist may put their hands on your mid-lower belly, a couple of creeps underneath your navel.

Position 9

Alternatively, an expert may offer Reiki to your knees and additionally to your lower legs or feet. These are discretionary positions if the specialist feels they may profit you. Or on the other hand, they may proceed onward to hand positions on your back.

Position 10

The specialist may ask for, on the off chance that you are on a back rub table, that you make over onto you feel sick with your head in face support or resting delicately to the other side. The specialist's hands are carefully put on your shoulder bone zone and rest there.

Position 11

Hands are descended to a situation under your cutting edges or center back.

Position 12

The expert moves their hands to apply delicate weight in a hand position at your lower back.

When the essential positions and additionally varieties have all been secured and stuck energies evacuated or adjusted, the specialist may move their hands over your body in a broad movement to purify your vitality field of any extra vitality flotsam and jetsam, leaving you washed down, feeling better, and well on your approach to upgraded prosperity.

**A while later**

It will be ideal if you make sure to drink a lot of water for 24 hours after your session and to take some time, even only two or three minutes, to delight in the serenity and quietness after your session. Attempt to permit 10 or 15 minutes at some point after your session or maybe later in the prior night bed to get thankfulness from your higher self for thinking about your body, brain, and soul and to make the most of your expanded condition of health and harmony.

# CHAPTER SIX

## AURA CLEANSING EXERCISES

The world wherein we live is three-dimensional, and it is comprised of vitality with various paces of vibration. Two sorts of dynamism impact air encompassing earth: the vitality of the universe, streaming downwards and the spirit of the planet, flowing upwards. The association of those energies makes up the vitality envelope of the earth, which empowers life to exist. Our body gets its required vitality for its right working from the vitality envelope of the planet. It is realized that an absence of parity in the atmosphere of the sun and the earth disturb life on earth. The sun - a goliath wellspring of vitality, transmits to all the Solar framework. While a sun overshadows, the radiation of energy is disturbed for a specific time, and touchy individuals feel the adjustment in the air.

We are in another age, the Age of Aquarius, which is not quite the same as the past age, Pisces. As of not long ago so as to create, we needed to raise the vitality from the earth upward. Today extraordinary sort of energy exists on earth. It originates from an alternate nearby planetary group. Presently we can get energy from above; however, for this, we should tune ourselves to it. This vitality is of incredible elegance. It impacts decidedly the atmosphere, opens the vitality channels, and changes the natural structure. There is a large inventory of light energy, which we can draw in.

Wellbeing and joy require the structure of the light around us - the air that encompasses us, and shields us from adverse impacts. Our very own light, our air, must be loaded up with immaculateness and the craving to carry satisfaction to people around us. We should work around us and inside us a stock of infinite vitality. We get it unreservedly. In reflection, we can send light to those needing it. It is fitting to stand quietly for a couple of minutes during the day, particularly before resting and clear the dirtied vitality in the emanation.

The universe comprises of seven levels where each level has its very own vibration. The seven degrees of cognizance is parallel to seven layers or bodies in man: the physical body, the essential body (enthusiastic), the astral body (sentiments), the psychological body (considerations), and the causal body (staying of the spirit). What's more, there is additionally an atmic body (level of the all-inclusive soul) and a monadic body (divine level).

Except for the physical body, every one of the bodies makes the Aura. In reality, the air is the electric and attractive radiation of the inconspicuous bodies. The emanation is an electromagnetic field, develop from vitality electrical cables. The electrical part is a level field, with its vitality lines orchestrated on a flat plane. The beautiful part is a vertical field, with its vitality lines organized vertically. Where the vitality is increasingly gathered in the atmosphere, vitality lines are made. The more lines an individual has, the more advantageous he is. When one stands in a vitality vacuum, for instance almost a TV, the lines shut down. Energy lines additionally exist around cells and organs — the electromagnetic field impacts personal satisfaction.

Prof. Harold Burr of Yale University depicted the atmosphere in the forties. He discovered that the physical body and the organs are worked from an electromagnetic field, and demonstrated that estimating the electromagnetic field of seed shows the potential development of the plant - shortcoming of the area identifies with issues in development. In 1910, Dr. Walter Kilner expounded on the vitality field of individuals and utilized shaded channels to demonstrate its reality. Dr. Wilhelm Reich, a specialist, later examined the connection between changes in the vitality of the body and the episode of physical and mental ailments. He was prevailing with regards to estimating the quality of the vitality field.

In this way, toward the start of the century, the atmosphere was at that point known. Sadly, even today, individuals are ignorant of its reality and impact on our wellbeing. The conventional drug doesn't perceive the quality, also though it thinks about the wonders of power in the body: With no power in the body and its organs, doctors couldn't utilize electrocardiogram or electroencephalogram – instruments that measure the ability in the heart and the cerebrum. Indeed, even single cells have electrical movement. During disease, there is a disturbance in the electromagnetic field and in the Bio-vitality stream. The physical body is the result of Bio-vitality - without Bio-vitality it degenerates.

The air is - as it were - our actual "article of clothing." It is comprised of light. We are a light emission, and any place we go the light of the Aura tails us. The body and the emanation retain and furthermore transmit vitality. Vitality is consistently in a powerful state, and every one of us communicates the vitality stream in one of a kind way. The quality ingests all the appropriate frequencies from the daylight. Here and there the air is splendid and extended, and once in a while, it is dull and contracted. We are sound when our breath is loaded with light, and there is no obstacle in the progression of vitality.

Our quality pulls in vitality from the environment, the sun and the moon, the blossoms, and other individuals. It works like a radio wire, which gets messages from the open world and the undetectable world.

The cleaner and more extensive the quality, the better is the gathering of a more noteworthy measure of impressions. The air assimilates misery or satisfaction, as indicated by its qualities. In the emanation, we see the state of our body and the nature of our contemplations and emotions. The light of the emission uncovers our character, transmits our pith, and ensures us. Its size is distinctive for every person. It is typically noticeable four-five feet outside the body, yet when the cognizance is consumed, it can arrive at ten feet or more. It is said that Buddha had a quality obvious for two miles.

The shades of the emanation are evolving immediately. In any case, radical changes don't usually happen inside a brief period. The atmosphere is comprised of various layers, and each layer has an alternate shading and shade. A few people have an extra-tactile visual perception, and they can see the shadows of the air. The shade of the imperative body, noticeable up to six crawls outside the physical body are blue-green. The shades of the astral body change always relying upon the feelings. Gold symbolizes the association with God and the affection for God. Brilliant hues show up with the improvement of profound awareness. At the point when the yellow shading shows up in the quality, it demonstrates mental movement. At the point when there is pink in the atmosphere, the individual transmits love. Violet express satisfaction, and green communicates development and abundance.

Dull yellow is the shade of scholarly vanity; dim red is the shade of enthusiasm. Hues are associated with sounds, and each stable has a fondness with a reasonable shading. Tones and hues can treat the air and help the mending and development of the body tissues. With age, the vitality in the body debilitates. Until the age of ten, it is packed in the lower some portion of the body-the tyke wants to run. At twenty the vitality arrives at its pinnacle and at eighty it is powerless, particularly in the lungs. Right breathing can ease the awful impacts of seniority, and on the off chance that we figure out how to inhale appropriately, we postpone maturing.

Various individuals have various emanations relying upon their contemplations and emotions, instruction, educational encounters, and karma. Each individual has an alternate pace of vibration, and every one of his issues is in actuality results of his considerations and emotions. In the event that an individual feelings of dread a mishap, he "draws towards himself " the misfortune due to his terror, because of his giving additional consideration to it. Profound improvement requires a defeating of negative sentiments that aggravate the existence of vitality and impact the air. Bliss is the result of an agreement between the bodies and the desire of the spirit. Each adjustment in the physical body relies upon the alteration in the vitality field and its pace of vibration. Individuals are not the same as one another by the splendor of the light, by the speed of the wave and by the shades of the atmosphere.

We worked inside us a great deal of worry, trying to limit our emotions and impulses. When we are irate or cry, the body shakes to express and discharge the distress or outrage. Outrage causes an expanded pulse and more prominent discharge of the organs. To release strain, we should express our sentiments in a controlled manner. When we are furious and neglect to express our displeasure, it collects inside our body and causes a blockage of vitality. The outcome is a difference in the shape and shade of the atmosphere. Each injury, enthusiastic stun, and damage causes a "jam" in the quality. We manufacture these "jams" as a guarded response, which irritates the entire vitality framework. When we experience an injury, we should yell or loosen up our hands and discharge strain. In the event that we can't scream, at that point, we should put our hands behind our back and victory air from the mouth energetically.

Ordinary prescription cases that by far most of all, sicknesses are psychosomatic, yet at the same time treats physical sickness for the most part in the soma (body) and once in a while in mind. We should regard the mind just as the body with the assistance of brain research, autosuggestion, day by day reflection, etc. There is a marvel called psycho-kinesis. It demonstrates that resolve can impact physical items. With the guide of psycho-kinesis, it is conceivable to move objects without contacting them. The intensity of will and the intensity of psyche are fundamental instruments. On the off chance that one can influence physical items, which are overwhelming and thick, with the utilization of the energy of will and the intensity of brain, one can likewise control emotions and considerations, which are subtler (not more fragile – simply subtler). We ought to figure out how to utilize self-control to impact the quality to avoid infection and to recoup from it.

Energy is to be found wherever known to humanity. It lights up us all, and we as a whole get it similarly. We get light on the off chance that we have the correct aim and on the off chance that we demand the light to add to people around us and not only for ourselves. We can twofold the size of the emanation on the off chance that we state multiple times boisterously: "I call the celestial Light; I am an ideal channel for the heavenly light. Light is the best direction for me". We ought to know that robust and iridescent air is our best security.

Ailment exists in the quality, a long time before it shows up in the physical body. While it is in the air, it can without much of a stretch be dealt with. Today, like never before, we should create preventive medication to counteract enduring and furthermore spare the immense cost spent on conventional drug. The air is a profound outline, which decides the soundness of the physical body. Ordinary medication ought to incorporate the atmosphere, the vitality focuses, and the energy diverts in its educating and practice.

As a rule, it is conceivable to forestall the advancement of ailments situated in the emanation by filtering feelings and considerations. Negative emotions and musings, and off-base and hurtful lifestyle, all make holes and shortcomings in the radiation, permitting the advancement of affliction. All that one does, each word the individual says, each idea, leave their engraving. On the off chance that the activities or considerations are sure and help our kindred people, the engravings stay constructive, and the individual pulls in and is encompassed by light. Along these lines, everybody manufactures his "sanctuary," his quality, and this way shapes his physical body.

Information about the quality causes us to know ourselves. There are various strategies to realize our vitality level and how to control it. Each cell in our body is a living insight and has the ability to deal with our body. The excellent administration of the cell relies upon the general equalization of the body. At the point when cells are not in parity, they stop to move the correct vibration and thus neglect to get from the mind the data about the right working. An individual can move vitality to cells denied of energy.

The exchange of energy invigorates the malignant cell to work. This innocuous activity is fundamental. It balances out the atmosphere and improves the vitality stream. At the point when the cell gets vitality, it can shield itself from microorganisms and infections. In the event that we recuperate others and ourselves, we additionally mend the aggregate electromagnetic field, which encompasses every one of us. This is simply an opportunity to know, to consider ourselves to be a vitality framework. We need to chip away at all levels - the mind, the psyche, and the spirit - since they are level of vitality that makes up the emanation. Issues at all levels are the aftereffect of need or excess of energy or stagnation of its stream, because of blockages in the vitality framework. The radiation of affection is the best radiation - love enlarges vitality; while abhor and misery decline it. When you emanate love, which has a place with the higher astral body in the quality, you can store the vitality of the sun inside you. When you are a piece of the highest energies of the universe, you can get instinct and Extra Sensory Perception.

After a decent rest, the atmosphere develops between four to six feet. The quality contracts during the day because of energy misfortune - particularly in the wake of visiting wiped out individuals or in the organization of individuals who draw a ton of vitality from us. On the off chance that you wish to move energy to other people, you ought to envision white light entering your head and your feet and leaving through your hands coordinated towards the individual. You should feel associated with the vitality.

We think we are autonomous, but then we are associated with the encompassing condition. Individuals with extra-tactile sight can see tracks - light bars discharged from vitality focuses. The tracks interface us as people. They uncover the sort of association and its quality. On the off chance that the connection between individuals isn't agreeable, the tracks are dull and clingy. A splendid string that interfaces the focuses of the core of two individuals demonstrate love. A string from the Solar plexus of one individual to the core of someone else reflects a desire to control sentiments. A string from the Solar plexus of the mother to the base of the spine of the youngster demonstrates an overbearing mother. In the connection between individuals, many strings are relying upon the quality and nature of the connections.

Emotions, considerations, discourse, and developments expend our vitality. Negative sentiments can hurt quality. At the point when two individuals come into shared contact, the combination of their airs is diverse depending on their emotions. It is realized that when two individuals are in closeness, there can be a condition of vitality similarity and their vitality fields commonly fortify one another. On the off chance that there is no similarity the vitality fields of the two people debilitate. It is conceivable to draw off vitality from the vitality field of someone else. The impact can be sure for one who additions energy and negative for the other who loses energy. On account of a couple where the man and the lady are good and corresponding in their vitality, they structure commonly an excellent vitality field, which coordinates and reinforces the couple.

All medications affect the air. Chemotherapy opens the emanation to negative impacts. The medical procedure leaves holes in the quality, which are destructive, and the patients are helpless for a few months. It is conceivable to treat the holes and the harmful impacts of medications by vigorous mending - by wrapping difficult spot with vitality. The back rub of agonizing spots additionally helps – the proposal is fifteen minutes of treatment for each spot. Each torment spot in the body is an emphasize point, and it ought to be discharged. For a situation of aggravation, - surplus vitality is concentrated and we need to draw off energy from the new spot. On the off chance that an organ is sick, at that point it doesn't emanate, and the atmosphere ends up dull.

During the recuperating procedure, the negative electrical field changes into a positive field and afterward returns to negative. Treatment with a negative vitality field accelerates recuperation time. Broken bones emanate negative flows. It is in this manner prescribed to stimulate the procedure by utilizing magnets, or with the guide of a current of negative particles. We are in charge of our atmosphere and should deal with it. Probably the ideal ways are to loosen up the body. It is prescribed to put the hand on the strained piece of the body and rationally loosen up it. In the event that the pressure doesn't leave the body, we first contract the muscles at that point unwind. When we are loosened up the cerebrum waves change, we get more vitality, and the energy focuses on opening up.

**How to Attract Energy to the Aura?**

Our body needs vitality to act. In the event that we need to be stable, we need to control the crucial energy, assimilate it proficiently and send it streaming in the body. It is conceivable to retain a lot of vitality by methods for rhythmical breathing and authority over our feelings and considerations. You can reinforce the air utilizing perception. Envision a white light that streams to you. Welcome and grasp the light. A short time later observe you encompassed in a white cloud. You ought to likewise attempt to detect the cloud, to feel how it nourishes every one of the cells and strokes your skin. In the event that we are adjusted genuinely, we can spare vitality. At the point when the body and soul are in agreement, the body takes care to deliver the fundamental energy. To be upbeat and to love increment body vitality. When you cherish, your quality is sparkling, and the more you adore and transmit love, people around you will improve. First, you should love yourself. To love yourself doesn't intend to manufacture and extend your inner self. Genuine romance "softens" the sense of self. The more you adore, the more you radiate the light vibration around you.

The emanation can be reinforced in unobtrusive ways, by tuning in to music, seeing tasteful items and by and large by making the most of our encompassing. We can impact the body cells with affection, energize them, and furthermore "tune in" to their reaction. We can emanate light to them. The Solar plexus is in charge of the imperativeness capacities, and when we are cheerful, the Solar plexus extends. You should fill it with light and tranquillity.

We ought to re-establish back to the emanation its positive hues and its unique sound. Great aromas and Aromatherapy are additionally useful. Etheric oils can carry energy to the radiation. The light of the full range is fundamental for our wellbeing and our spirit. Glaring light is hurtful to prosperity, and it is along these lines better to utilize incandescent lamp secured with glass. It is likewise prescribed to place shells, precious stones, blooms and plants in the parlour, yet not in the room. It is conceivable to impact the emanation with aromas and hues, with Bach blossoms, with the drinking of pearl elixirs. Open to the sun a gem in liquor or water for quite a while until the fluid assimilates the vibration of the precious stone. You can utilize a hued glass presented to the sun to get a particular shading in the quality. Singing changes, the mind waves and has a positive impact on the emanation. It is magnificent to sing while at the same time, having a shower. The water cleans the body, and the sound sweeps the cynicism from the air.

You ought to recollect that we came here to this world to fabricate an assortment of light. It is imperative to adore ourselves because a low mental self-portrait drains the vitality in the atmosphere. In a workshop, we checked the size of the emanation when we envisioned that we are increasing and more grounded. After representation, we found a more prominent and increasingly clear atmosphere. The body and the psychological procedures need vitality. The most significant nourishment is the vitality, which enters through breathing, particularly during rest. Swimming in the ocean does some incredible things, and you exploit both the sun and saltwater which clean the body and thus it can twofold the size of the quality.

Additionally, mud showers include vitality. It is prescribed to be in nature, at any rate, a couple of hours consistently. To keep up excellent wellbeing perception of swimming in a perfect and splendid shading goodly affects the quality. Utilize orange for essentialness, green for development, blue for tranquillity, and violet for virtue. Reflection develops the air and interfaces us with new elements of mindfulness. On the off chance that you picture that you are lying on the shoreline and retain into the stomach, the beams of a warming sun – you bit by bit will feel the glow. You can likewise feel how the waves bring light into your body, and as they haul out, they clean all pessimism. On the off chance that moreover, you recall happy occasions, you will feel much improved, and this positive sentiment will be reflected in the air. In this condition, the brain produces alpha waves, and the electromagnetic field demonstrates 7.5 cycles every second - the vigorous condition in reverberation with the recurrence of the Earth. In the event that we understand that we are otherworldly fundamentally, we can extend our emanation and grow our mindfulness.

We are associated with God and the universe through our spirit, which uses the lower bodies to accomplish its objective. In the event that you like to raise your pace of vibration, you can utilize purple plates1. These plates transmit positive vitality when setting under plants or on the agonizing spot. It is prescribed to put nourishment and water fifteen minutes on the plates. The water is additionally useful for watering plants. The plates kill the antagonism in nourishment and water and furthermore change the flavour of the wine. For whatever length of time that you keep them in your emanation – in a pocket or a tote, you will feel an expansion of vitality. To adjust the energy, you can likewise utilize "Miniaturized scale Crystal Cards." These are produced using a material created by NASA to wrap round the team lodge and kill the negative impacts of the room. With an electrochemical procedure minute, estimated gems are carved into the Micro Crystal Card. Individuals utilizing them can adjust the negative energies that are available in their vitality field. Purple plates, Micro Crystal plates, Bach blooms, and precious stones can help us, particularly on the off chance that we are prepared to refine our feelings and musings. We can enhance the emanation and make it more brilliant by our emotions - with adoration, tolerance, petition, positive reasoning, and furthermore by helping other people to create constructive characteristics. The characteristics of virtue, unselfishness, quietude, and confidence can improve our character. Inward chip away at our integrity, improvement of positive characteristics, and disposing of negative traits are in every case more potent than outer treatment. By inner work, we can improve our lifestyle and change our fate.

For what reason is it so imperative to treat the emanation? A lovely and splendid air pulls in magnificence and immaculateness, though a dim and ruined quality draws in contamination. A dirty air can't shield us and can't get messages from the higher universes. At the point when the etheric, astral and mental bodies are unadulterated, we draw in and ingest more vitality and better impressions. Kindly remember that creatures from higher universes see our emanation and not our physical body. It doesn't make a difference in what we do, and it is in every case great to know about our atmosphere. When getting up toward the beginning of the day or before resting it is a great idea to envision that a ball loaded with light encompasses us from the feet up to the head and that our body, particularly our heart is sparkling.

We ought to recall that snickering light up the atmosphere and is infectious, so we ought to recollect exciting events, take a gander at an image of a grinning face, encircle ourselves with giggling individuals and make individuals chuckle.

### How Might We See the Aura?

A strategy has been created to photo the air, and it is called Kirlian photography. Nicola Tesla and the Kirylian couple built up this method of photography. By and large, everybody can figure out how to see the air. On the off chance that you like to know the atmosphere, you should initially do breathing activities. The point is to revive the action of the body and carry more vitality to the body frameworks, including the eyes. A short time later, eye works out. Roll the eyes right and left, here and there and around. This activity improves the muscles of eyes, reinforce the eyes, and accelerate the movement of the poles in the eye that see haziness and light and the cones that see essential hues yellow, blue and red. We utilize just a piece of the light that enters the eyes. Clairvoyants utilize 35% of the light in vision, and a great many people utilize 15-20% The more vitality comes through the eye to the nerve, the better we see.

The accompanying activity is vital: Stretch the hand forward and place the finger at the tallness of the eye. On the off chance that you need to see the air of the finger look at the finger, without centering, move it in reverse and advances while taking a gander at it all the time in a casual manner. The emanation can likewise be seen with uncommon glasses*. In any case, before utilizing them, you need to practice the eye muscles to create more exceptional affectability to the correlative hues. Take a gander at a hued surface under a substantial light, red for instance, and a while later close the eyes or take a gander at a white sheet of paper. At that point, you will see the corresponding shading green. Do these multiple occasions. The activity to see the corresponding hues is useful. I saw the quality round the fingers when they were laid on a dull surface, and one hand contacted the other. When I put the fingers further away, I found in the space between the fingers the air of the fingers. This demonstrates the emanation moves more gradually than the body.

You can attempt the accompanying analysis: sit in a faintly lit room, loosen up the body and take a gander at a man remaining beside a white divider. Take a gander at him without centering - along these lines, you can see the crucial body. In the event that a man rapidly hops aside, you can see the essential air on the divider, after he has moved away. This trial likewise demonstrates that the air moves in a slower rate than the body, yet despite everything, it pursues the developments of the body a similar way. Now and then, the emanation isn't adjusted appropriately with the physical body. After encountering injury, fears, it can move advances, in reverse or sideward and doesn't come back to the suitable spot. This makes sick impacts, and man doesn't feel well – as goes the well-known axiom: "he isn't inside his skin."

Today it is conceivable to photo the atmosphere with an exceptional Polaroid camera. You can figure out how to see the quality, yet it is anything but difficult to figure out how to detect it. How might we sense the air? The palm of the hand, measured like a bowl, is like a radio wire dish, and it can analyze various frequencies. The vast majority feel vitality as warmth, cold, or a shivering sensation. A healer is an individual who feels the progression of energy. To detect energy, place the hand over the TV or the PC screen, close the eyes and gradually bring down the hand over the outside of the screen at short of what one and a half inches away. In the event that you don't feel the vitality, maybe the reason is that the hand isn't loosened up enough or it isn't touchy. You can ignore the hands' plants and hues to feel the distinctions in the vibe of the hand.

An important exercise to detect vitality is to "fabricate" a vitality ball with the assistance of the hands. In this activity, it is significant that the spine is straight. To animate the feeling of vitality, carry vitality to the hands by scouring them, shaking them, boxing then again. Move the hands measured before you a few times to shape a non-existent ball, until you feel the opposition noticeable all around. Thereafter you let the hands along the edge of the body to feel the progression of vitality. On the off chance that you draw close to an individual and your hands are delicate to energy, you feel the obstruction of his emanation. Numerous years prior, I embraced a thought from a profound man. He prompted me to make an "inflatable" and engrave a desire, whatever I might want to occur, in it. The "expand" we provide for the general soul, who chooses as indicated by the inestimable laws if to understand this desire or to surrender it.

## How to Cleanse the Aura?

Different electrical apparatuses: TV's, PCs, and so forth., make friction based electricity that adheres to the atmosphere, contaminates it and avoids vitality to experience it. Moreover, our negative considerations and sentiments, and the negative musings of others towards us taint the quality. In addition to the fact that we need to clean the physical body, yet we likewise need to scrub the electromagnetic field, which influences the physical body. We can purify quality in various ways. Here is one approach to purge it: the advisor remains inverse the patient. He puts his hands over the leader of the patient and moves them from the head to the feet multiple times back, numerous times forward, and numerous times to the sides. He shakes hands each time he moves his hands from the head to the feet to dispose of the build-up of negative vitality. When the treatment, the advisor must wash his hands up to the elbows. It is conceivable to clear, to strip the atmosphere by little developments of the hands and to envision that a "vacuum cleaner" is sucking up the soil. The hands ought to be shaken toward the part of the arrangement. Next, the air is accused of clean vitality. The accusing is completed of the positive hand.

Another technique tends to three levels:

The bones - the purifying is finished by passing a measured hand from head to toes with long and

Consistent developments for five minutes. The separation is eight crawls from the body.

The blood framework - The development is clockwise a good way off of sixteen crawls from the body, and it is finished with a level hand for three minutes.

The nerves - The developments of the fingers are sharp and short, copying piano playing. The separation is twenty creeps from the body and the time-one moment.

The treatment is given with no contact with the patient and with the accepting hand (with a great many people, it's the left palm). It is a great idea to have blossoms close by to toss the contaminated vitality on them. The blooms exist on a lower vitality level, and dirtied energy for us nourishes them. You can likewise purge the quality with precious stones or consume salvia (a recuperating herb) and enable the smoke to fold over the body. Absorbing the legs for ten minutes of water with ocean salt elevates the body vibration and cleans the lower vitality focuses. It is a great idea to have a shower with ocean salt and soft drink powder. You can likewise rub the body, particularly agonizing joints with this blend.

Tibetan cymbals are an extra technique for cleaning the emanation. The development of the cymbals is from the highest point of the body towards the base sideways, forward lastly in reverse. Everybody can do this for himself. The cymbals can likewise clean the air in the workplace and at home. On the off chance that you need to dispose of any torment or to sully in a specific piece of the body, place the accepting hand a good way off of two creeps from the excruciating territory. Make hovers over the spot and draw out the sullied vitality. Haul out your hand some good ways off from the emanation and fold it to dispose of the contaminated energy. Envision discarding the contamination far into the ground, if there are no blooms or plants close by to retain it.

By and large, it is sufficient to clean the quality to improve wellbeing. Despondency and awful mind-sets frequently are the consequences of amassing of patches of electricity produced via friction in the air. It is essential to recall that there is no reason for moving vitality without first cleaning the atmosphere. On the off chance that the emanation is filthy, it won't enable new energy to infiltrate. Cleaning is the principal thing one ought to do. To ensure the atmosphere, we envision a huge chime covering us, or we can likewise envision a chunk of white or blue light around us. We can likewise inhale light through the legs and head and load up with light the air during exhalation. The atmosphere can be intentionally pulled in towards the body when we be less helpless against outside powers.

In the focal pivot of the body there is an etheric channel called Antahkarana. It joins us with Earth and Heaven, with our spirit and higher measurements. The Antahkarana is the focal channel of a Pillar of Light, which encompasses us. Imagining the Pillar of Light and the Antahkarana carries agreement to the emanation and secure us. We are altogether made of vitality fields, which impact different creatures and things around us. The person is a little piece of a more noteworthy quintessence. It is the gathering spot of various energies, a reality that the mind discovers hard to fathom. Individuals are prepared to practice for the wellness their physical body. What are they prepared to accomplish for the wellness of their emanation, which is really in charge of the strength of the physical body?

The following are works out, which fortify the air. While practicing it is critical to feel the contact with the ground, and envision that the feet have progressed toward becoming roots that enter somewhere down in the ground. By establishing ourselves we get the vitality of the earth. By establishing we adjust the vitality focuses of the body which causes us carry the light into the whole body.

Exercise No. 1

Remain in the situation of Tai Chi – marginally bowed the knees to permit the progression of vitality starting from the earliest stage, shoulders are dropped and the tongue contacts the sense of taste. Inhale profoundly through the stomach. After the inward breath hold the breath, delicately tighten the butt and the frontal sphincter five seconds (the check from one to five) and afterward unwind by smothering the air. Do this activity a few times as it builds the ability to assimilate, hold, and discharge vitality.

Exercise No. 2 - The picture of the egg

You can envision the air as an egg of amazing white light, which step by step augments. Feel that by developing and extending it builds the light. From the start the light spreads out from the focal point of the heart. Feel that the heart transmits vitality, imagine that the emanation is spreading to around ten feet on each side of the body and afterward it develops to the size of the room, the size of the nation, the size of the earth and in the long run the size of the universe. At that point the other way lessen the quality to its common size. It is ideal to do this activity with rhythmical relaxing.

Exercise No. 3 - The Thread of Life

Envision a loop thirty crawls in measurement, which is folded over you, it starts from the feet and goes up clockwise. It throbs with a violet fire, which reinforces the air. In the wake of inclination OK with the development, picture a comparative loop, which goes around a counter clockwise way. First and foremost, do the development independently. Later on proceed with the two developments simultaneously. It is essential to encounter a clockwise development that draws in vitality to the middle and a counterclockwise development that transmits vitality outwards. It is additionally great to envision yourself inside a segment loaded up with violet light with a defensive white wrapping. Violet, the shade of the flame, has sanitizing properties. Attempt to feel that a violet flame expends the physical and mental contamination and leaves you sanitized.

Exercise No. 4

Remain on one foot, move the hands downwards and upward a few times in front and the sides of the body with the palms of the hands measured and confronting the floor. Keep on moving the hands in mood. Attempt to feel the air drag. A short time later change the position and remain on the other leg. Proceed with the developments. After some time, attempt to "pull" the air - loosen up your hands gradually toward each path in a cadenced manner with a measured palm. Feel the air obstruction when you outstretch the hands. Do this activity with Ravel's "Bolero" which is rhythmical music? The activity catches the earth attraction.

Exercise No. 5 - The segment of Light

Stand completely loose and envision that you are in a segment of six feet in measurement. It shields you from each external impact. Inhale profoundly and find in your creative mind how the section is loaded up with an orange shading with each breath. The whole body produces orange vitality and it fills the segment with this vitality. Envision following five moments a white light pouring on you. It covers you and brings genuine feelings of serenity. Envision daylight on the navel, which warms your body. Carry the daylight to the heart, feel how the heart transmits love and fill the air with light. State so anyone might hear, "I am produced using light, I serve the light and the light resuscitates me, ensures me, guides me and recuperates me." This significant exercise refines, pairs the size of the air, and fills us with energy.

There are different activities, which reinforce the emanation including various types of breath, Tai Chi, Chi Kung activities and Yoga stances. To hop on a trampoline initiates, the progression of the cerebrospinal liquid and is another approach to get vitality. Keep in mind that whenever you need security, you may request that Archangel Michael encompass you with his blue light and to cut with his sword every one of the tracks that predicament you.

# CHAPTER SEVEN

## HOW TO INCREASE YOUR LIFE FORCE ENERGY

A Reiki specialist channels general life-power energy to recuperate, more often than not through the palms of the hands. Furthermore, as indicated by Mikao Usui, Reiki's author, specialists can transmit Reiki mending through the hands as well as through "any piece of the physical body"; the delicate look or delicate breath of an expert who develops consciousness of Reiki's unobtrusive vitality can be as recuperating as the bit of Reiki-charged hands.

This capacity to channel general life-power vitality sets Reiki separated from both antiquated recuperating customs and other current modalities. For instance, Reiki contrasts from "laying on of hands," with which it is regularly looked at, in that it doesn't require either the "healer" or the beneficiary of recuperating to have confidence of any sort. Individuals all things considered, just as freethinkers and nonbelievers, can and do learn Reiki and practice it viably on their customers; individuals everything being equal, just as skeptics and agnostics, can and do get Reiki medications and experience magnificent mending benefits. Reiki essentially works, on devotees and non-adherents

the same. Reiki is additionally not normal for shamanism, which has been polished for a large number of years in ancestral societies. This antiquated, noteworthy custom requires the healer to assume the infection of the individual needing recuperating all together for that individual to turn out to be free of disease. Reiki doesn't require taking on any other person's physical ailment, mental anguish, or enthusiastic misery. Rather, both the Reiki expert and the customer get some recuperating, in spite of the fact that the customer who is the planned beneficiary encounters by a wide margin the best mending impacts.

Reiki is additionally unmistakable from some cutting edge recuperating modalities, for example,

Swedish back rub, which require the expert to work the customer's strained muscles into a progressively loosened up state. Reiki doesn't physically assessment or fumes a specialist, on the grounds that no physical exertion, other than setting the hands in position, is expected to channel the recuperating vitality. However numerous customers will remark, toward the part of the bargain treatment, "That was superior to a back rub." They have felt the calming impacts of the energy so profoundly that they snapped off and after that arose totally loose and invigorated. To be sure, knead specialists and physical advisors regularly learn Reiki with the goal that they can offer their customers a mending methodology that doesn't, finished

time, stress their very own muscles and ligaments to the point of carpal passage disorder. Increasingly more authorize back rub schools offer Reiki among their course postings. Since the Reiki technique for common recuperating uses directed vitality of a higher power, the specialist's energies are not depleted. Truth be told, most Reiki specialists guarantee that doing a treatment makes them feel "energized." This is a result of the progression of the vitality itself. It streams into the professional first, to carry mending and help to any region of worry in the specialist's body, and afterward it moves through the expert's hands to the customer. Like within a nursery hose, which stays adaptable and in great condition when it is utilized regularly to water parched ground, the expert advantages from the progression of vitality that courses into her and through her. Numerous individuals feel that the hands they bring to Reiki are now "mending hands." Massage specialists, medical attendants, specialists, chiropractors—without a doubt, anybody—can deliberately work with symbolism, attestation, and expectation to fortify the recuperating character of their hands. Reiki incredibly upgrades whatever regular or developed recuperating capacity an understudy has; if the understudy feels he has no common mending capacity, Reiki sets up without question that the understudy has been invested with the capacity to channel a higher request of recuperating power.

The main physical exertion that the individual Reiki specialist needs to make is to put his hands some place—on himself, on a customer on the treatment table, around an earthenware pot holding a lemon-scented geranium—and the mending vitality will stream voluntarily. For whatever length of time that the Reiki specialist has been appropriately receptive to channel the recuperating vitality, at that point he need not be focused or grounded or profoundly elevated or even feeling great. When he puts his hands down, the Reiki vitality will stream—and the experience of directing this mending vitality will focus and ground and elevate and carry recuperating to the Reiki specialist, just as to the individual, the creature, the plant under his hands.

This is one of the incredible advantages of learning conventional Usui Reiki: by only collaborating with the vitality stream, the specialist realizes his own recuperating. This is one reason that Reiki professionals don't call themselves "healers." They are very much aware that the all-inclusive life-power vitality is the genuine healer and does all the genuine work of recuperating.

## The Breathing Process

To inhale is to get life power, and to expand our very own vitality. Great breathing carries with it most extreme vitality through least exertion. The vast majority don't inhale appropriately. A total cycle of breathing is worked in three stages. At the principal stage, the Solar plexus and the stomach ascend, as we push out our tummy and fill our lungs with air. Putting the palms of the hands on the stomach, to check its developments, is prescribed. The lower some portion of the lungs is topped off, first, at that point the lungs center part, and right a short time later the upper part. At the subsequent stage, we stop the relaxing for five seconds - that is the time required for the essential vitality, which is noticeable all around, to arrive at the platelets. Short breathing would not pass on to the blood its essentialness. The more we keep the air in our lungs, the more wellbeing and vitality we get. In the wake of holding our breath, breathing out is done considerably more proficiently. At the third stage we breathe out the air through the nose, in a very inverse manner to the breathing in procedure. We push the ribs with the neckline bone downwards, and push the gut muscles internal to breathe out all the caught air. These activities ought to be performed normally, without power.

Breathing is a characteristic procedure, without strain and exertion. The most ideal approach to practice it is by lying on the floor - or by sitting with feet held tight together, and the jaw held forward, so as to fix the spine. Researchers have discovered that during a full, profound breathing, the mind emanates progressively Alpha waves, and that causes unwinding. Ten minutes of cognizant, profound breathing, fills us with vitality and tranquillity. It is an activity that dissuades strain and dread. By holding our breath, cells get more oxygen, on account of the more drawn out span of contact with the air. We may see through visionary vision, that during the time the breath is held, a tremendous measure of Prana is spread in the body - that never happens when we don't hold our breath. An increasingly proficient approach to hold our breath is by getting the sphincters (the butt and the frontal sphincter).

When we are getting the sphincters we contract our stomach too, and that helps particularly the breathing procedure. It is constantly prescribed to pull the stomach inside while breathing out. The breathing ought to consistently be done through the nose as the air heats up, along these lines killing contrasts of temperature, between the body and nature. The hairs of the nose additionally channel out residue and earth particles that may cause aggravations. Air incorporates nitrogen, oxygen, and Prana - life's vitality. These components are blended with one another, however Prana can go through dividers, and is found all over. There is no spot without Prana. To get it by breathing is basic. We hold Prana in a few structures:

- Through the tips of the nose's nerves.
- Through the tongue which uncovers the preference for nourishment - and that is the reason biting is so significant.
- Through the skin in remaining under the daylight.
- Through breathing through the air.
- Through the eyes.

- Through representation and focus. These expand the amount of the Prana.

Prana complies with the voice of the idea. When breathing is under cognizant control, we can hold more Prana.

The majority of the otherworldly healers accentuate the significance of breathing, in profound advancement. Accusing the blood of oxygen and Prana is a key to modify and mend the physical body. When we don't inhale all around ok, harms collect, the body's vibration diminishes, and there is a negative effect on body and soul. While we develop, we neglect to inhale appropriately. Shallow breathing, just with the development and compression of the lungs, without the development of the stomach, doesn't permit unwinding.

In each breath that we take, the universe conveys air into us, and siphons it back when we breathe out it. Breathing discloses to us that we are a piece of the soul that works everything. In Buddhism, the beat of breathing is being utilized to grow the outskirts of the Ego. When you inhale, attempt to know to the all-inclusive energy - and do express gratitude toward it, for vitalizing each cell in your body - and you will get the world inside yourself. When you breathe out, send your much obliged, your vitality, to all the enduring individuals. Consequently, you get life by breathing in, and you give from yourself by breathing out. Breathing in speaks to the likelihood to get, and breathing out speaks to the give up, the giving, and carries with it unwinding. Breathing is a common component to both body and soul. It is an activity that widens our cognizance. It is a great idea to envision that the air climbs along the spine, when we breathe out, and slide along it when we breathe in.

The air we breathe in makes certain progressions inside us, and afterward gets out. We should give it a chance to get out. On the off chance that we won't breathe out the air, we would not have the option to get new and natural air. On the off chance that we wish to get during our lives, we need to give. On the off chance that we include kept inside ourselves sentiments of outrage, of aspiration, or negative emotions - we can give them a chance to out by the activity of breathing out. Along these lines, we empower life vitality to stream inside - while the poisons are being let out of the body. So as to get the grandiose vitality - the widespread power we need to inhale intentionally, to breathe in the light and the excellence and to cast out by breathing out the fiendishness, the malady and the dread. We are breathing deliberately when with each breathing in we associate with the universe and with each exhalation we send light and love to the earth.

To inhale appropriately the spine must be straight. It is conceivable to see the body's degree of vitality through the stance of the chest. Enthusiastic pressure makes the chest solidify. Negative emotions solidify the chest, which causes breathing issues and absence of vitality. We should treat the solidified chest, loosen up the emotions (a psychological procedure), and work on the chest's stance (a physical procedure). The chest will permit the passage of substantially more air, and more vitality, when it is adaptable and discharged. A "shield" in the chest territory, or the Solar plexus, demonstrates that the individual is loaded with wrath, and expects to do brutal action. At that point issues of stomach, respiratory framework or the liver and nerve bladder may show up.

Cognizant breathing empowers legitimate contemplation and decidedly impacts our wellbeing, while fixation on the entry of air through the nostrils brings more Prana to the body. We more often than not inhale twelve times each moment; during contemplation we inhale multiple times or even less every moment - yet in a lot further way. During reflection, we loosen up the body. At the point when the body is loose, there is a decent progression of vitality if there have not been blockages for an all-inclusive time. When we focus on our breathing, day by day issues are overlooked and intrusions of the external world disappear step by step - while this movement calms the contemplations, and empowers us to tune in to our body. In the event that we focus on a specific thing, and get eager, or on the off chance that we feel a forceful passionate fervor or dread, we quit relaxing. When we start breathing, once again, we for the most part quickly swallow the air. A fundamentally the same as thing happens when we eat excessively quick. The outcome is gas and stomachaches. In this manner it is essential to show ourselves how not to quit breathing, and how to inhale appropriately.

Breathing mirrors our state of mind, and equally it may change our mind-set. When we are upbeat we inhale profoundly, and when we cry, the body is twisted and we take in short and sporadic fits. Power over breathing empowers authority over emotions.

As per Dr. Drunvalo Melchizedek, an etheric direct exists in the body for the progression of Prana inside us - it is two creeps in distance across, its length from eight crawls underneath our feet, up to somewhere in the range of eight creeps over our heads. Man used to inhale from the outset through that channel, while concentrating the vitality of the earth and the universe in a certain chakra. In such a breathing procedure the Prana would go through the pineal organ and actuate it. The pineal organ would get the vitality and circulate it all through the body. This organ associates us with the binding together head of the universe. Today, in view of changes in the breathing procedure, we don't utilize that organ any longer. It did therapist and we presently get the duality of the universe rather than the solidarity. Dr. Melchizedek prescribes breathing and drawing the Prana from the universe and the earth through the etheric channel, gathering it from the start in the Solar plexus, later in the Heart's chakra and from that point transmit it into the emanation. The Prana radiation in addition to unlimited love elevate us to higher circles.

Why we prescribe to inhale further and all the more gradually? In the event that we inhale gradually, we can avert outrage. Outrage and dread, which cause pressure, accelerate the breathing procedure in an undesirable manner. Notwithstanding when there are sentiments of dread and stress, we should inhale appropriately. Especially during stress periods, we should inhale gradually - the propensity for tallying up to ten preceding any further advance helps in instances of pressure. Dread when all is said in done and stage trepidation might be defeated through moderate relaxing. We inhale around ten to twelve times each moment. When we take in a shallow way, we decline the ingestion of vitality, and we don't broaden the lungs' volume. The result is firm lungs; and thus, profound breathing would be uncommon and difficult to perform, and out of the accessible vitality we would utilize just a little part. At the point when torments attack us, we need to inhale profoundly and focus on the breath, not to the agony. This sort of movement doesn't dispose of the torment, yet can lessen it.

Focus reinforces everything on which we concentrate. That is the reason it is a great idea to figure out how to focus on breathing, notwithstanding the agony. Without an air loaded with particles we can't endure. The particle's state is a state, wherein the dynamic molecule may give or get an electron. Positive particles effectively retain electrons and negative particles are prepared to give electrons. It is charming to inhale almost a cascade or in a woodland or just after a tempest - when the quantity of negative particles noticeable all around is high. Then again, before a tempest we feel a substantial burden noticeable all around, due to the colossal amount of positive particles in it. At home the circumstance isn't perfect for solid breathing, because of the incredible measure of electronic gadgets, for example, TVs, PCs, radios, notwithstanding rugs, backdrop and fabrics made of manufactured material, which produce positive particles. In the cutting edge period, the measure of negative particles in the city is decreased as these particles hold fast to clean, smoke scents and tobacco, and tumble to the ground. The convergence of negative particles increases our sharpness, hinders the breathing procedure and realizes a positive sentiment, helping our focus. The air that we for the most part inhale is stacked with a negative burden, whiles the air that we breathe out is stacked with emphatically charged carbon oxide.

We suggest utilizing an ionizer which cleans the sullied air in workplaces, homes, autos and particularly in smoking zones. It is essential to know about the way that the atmosphere contains particles, similarly as the body is made of iotas. The electrons are particles of light, and inside our body the progression of negative particles inside the cells, blesses us with life - because of the digestion and the breathing procedure.

Breathing interfaces body and soul as it is the body's just programmed capacity that can be effectively changed through cognizant will. Breathing brings oxidation and empowers organ work. Do the breathing in through the nose, yet imagine that it is done through the arms and legs and the Root chakra. Carry the air to the Hara region. Every one of those breathings, which gather much vitality at the Hara, may invigorate fervor and even tremors - if the vitality isn't utilized toward the part of the arrangement. The vitality is scattered by envisioning how it circles multiple times the navel clockwise, and multiple times the other way, counter clockwise - that is the means by which it works with men, and the other way around with ladies. This breathing brings vitality everywhere throughout the body. With training you can learn through perception to inhale through the bones, the skin or any organ for fortifying.

**Incomprehensible Breathing**

While breathing in draw the tummy inside and contract the Solar plexus, which moves descending and makes weight on the organs in its region.

Simultaneously the vitality is being moved to the meridians. While breathing out enlarge the volume of the stomach region, by exploding the paunch. The procedure is inverse to common relaxing. Essentialness tops off the Hara zone. This sort of breathing is utilized while rehearsing Chi-Kung and Tai Chi. Yoga educators guarantee this is the correct method for relaxing.

## Cooling Breathing

We load the body with positive vitality by breathing; we quiet it and loosen up it. It is conceivable to heat up or to cool the body, by breathing and focusing on it. It is conceivable to change the Prana – the grandiose vitality, into a sentiment of warmth or cool, as per the condition of breathing in. Inhale profoundly with legs consolidated, and envision that with each breath the air is cooled. Similarly, you can heat up the body, yet most importantly you should gather in an exceptionally little piece of the body. Another technique to cool the body is by reaching out a piece of the tongue - a large portion of an inch – and collapsing it into a U shape, similar to a bow. The breathing is done through the tongue while it is in the state of a sickle; we at that point hold our breath and breathe out through the nose. The air in conventional breathing enters through the nose and makes warmth in that manner; while in this technique, it enters through the mouth and makes coolness. Taking along these lines accelerates digestion and has great effect on the eyes, ears and the liver.

**Breathing Through the Energy Centers**

Breathing through the energy focuses is conceivable, and breathing through the Solar plexus or the Hara focus is prescribed specifically. The breathing is performed through the lungs, however simply envision that it is done through the energy focuses. You may inhale the sun's energy or the world's energy.

The technique depends on a hypothesis' case that vitality is coordinated to wherever, by idea and the correct practice. Put your hands on the main vitality focus while you envision when breathing in the red shading. Feel how the inside is topped off with vivid Prana when you hold your breath - and afterward breathe out. Do it a few times with each vitality focus, and its correct shading. Toward the end, so as to interface the vitality focuses one to the next, envision that you breathe in the Prana from your feet to the main vitality focus, and a short time later, from the principal focus to the subsequent one, etc. through every one of the focuses.

**An Additional Exercise**

It is a blend of breathing activities with representation. You should attempt to find in your imagination how the air enters the body. Feel how it streams inside your body, and warms you, how it fills the body's organs. Envision that with the air the heavenly love, which is all over the place, enters in your body. When you hold your breath, feel how it fills each cell in your body. While breathing out, send forward your hands, with broadened and open fingers and feel how you emanate love to the universe. It is a great idea to envision that each breath joins you with the universe. After the breathing activities it is a lot simpler to feel the progression of vitality - the warmth, the sensitive sentiments and vibrations in the arms.

## A Breathing Exercise That Loads the Body with Energy

Inhale and envision the vitality ingestion. Breathe in, hold your breath and keeping in mind that breathing out, send the vitality by representation to the agonizing territory or organ through your hands. In the second time that you hold your breath, feel as though the vitality is entering the excruciating organ. Breathing activities with perception are utilized for mending. Seeing the natural air that transmits the vitality to the blood, in an individual's imagination - is very attractive. Feel how the activity is accomplished in the body. When you are breathing in, envision your contemporary state - your harmed cells for example; and when you hold your breath think about the message and the image that would actuate the cells of a particular organ. Somewhere in the range of three seconds are typically satisfactory for it, however time may be enlarged. At that point request the capacities to be done while breathing out, imagining how the breath dives deep into every cell of the harmed organ.

When breathing in the counsel is to "welcome" the light, "breath" the light; and keeping in mind that breathing out to send it to the organs, to some harmed region, or to the universe. Focus on the light, and send it to everybody. Along these lines you discharge a solid otherworldly vitality that raises the human awareness. It is critical to recall that common breathing is normal and programmed, and is managed with no exertion. The activities are an instrument that causes us arrive at the correct method to relax. Profound and appropriate breathing can improve our wellbeing, correct our feelings and carry with it positive sentiment, unwinding and significant serenity. It would be a pity, not to adventure such a basic and regular procedure that has inside it such huge numbers of potential outcomes.

**Sustenance**

With legitimate sustenance we add a very long time to our life, with terrible nourishment we abbreviate our life. The nourishment we eat affects our physical and psychological wellness. Truly we are what we digest, as each cell in our body is made from the sustenance we eat. Awful wellbeing is the result of three principle

**Factors:**

1. Collection of toxic substances in the body, as a result of an ill-advised eating regimen.
2. Absence of supplements as a result of eating prepared and rationed sustenance.
3. Stress and negative musings and sentiments.

**Sustenance Absorption**

Numerous individuals don't know that absorption begins in the mouth. The stomach related procedure begins with the smell, the sight, even the idea of sustenance. Hence, it is imperative to bite the sustenance well, plant it into minor particles, and accordingly facilitate the absorption procedure. Like the human body, sustenance also has biochemical and electromagnetic vitality, and biting discharges the vitality inside it. As per Indian prescription we need to bite the sustenance thirty-two times. The point is to process the sustenance and transform it nearly into a fluid, and after that to swallow it. The demonstration of biting discharges the salivation, which helps absorption. It isn't prescribed to eat and drink simultaneously, however to drink between dinners - clear water would be the best. It is prescribed to have sustenance in its dry structure, since drinking fluids with eating nourishment weakens the gastric fluids.

When we are anxious and eat excessively quick, we don't process appropriately. Before eating inhale profoundly a few times and loosen up the body, feel the congruity that exists among you and the nourishment and offer thanks as it is acclimated in various religions. As indicated by the assessment of dietitians, adjusted nourishment is made out of half - 60% starches; 20% protein, which is significant for tissue development and support; 30% of fat - separated into 20% of unsaturated fat and 10% of soaked fat. A protein-enhanced eating routine bombshells absorption, and furthermore irritates the activity of the heart and kidneys. Immersed fats cause courses blockages. It is in this manner prescribed to diminish the utilization of domesticated animal's items, meat and entire milk, which contain immersed fat. Our body helps us to remember a vehicle. The starches and the fat are the body's fuel and oil, however without the electric sparkle - the vitality, the vehicle won't begin. To our lament individuals tend their autos more than their own bodies. They never put water rather than fuel in their vehicle's tank, however they continue eating prepared nourishment, which incorporates extra fixings that the body can't process. The body can adapt as long as it has a reasonable hold of vitality and proteins, yet insusceptibility doesn't keep going forever.

So as to ease processing, it is prescribed not to blend strong sustenance of various supplements. In this way proteins (meat) ought not be blended with starches (batter and bread). Organic products ought to be eaten crisp, and we should hold up twenty - thirty minutes before eating whatever else. It is smarter to set up the supper directly before gobbling it in light of the fact that continued heating up of sustenance and continued cooling in the icebox - diminishes its sustaining esteem. With respect to sweet nourishments, they ought to be totally relinquished (aside from nectar), likewise industrialized sustenance, which contains substance fixings. Bugs are more effective than men. On the off chance that we have for example two packs of flour, - crude flour, and white flour – the bugs will favor the crude flour that contains minerals.

## All Encompassing Healing

All-encompassing recuperating means re-establishing wholeness and blessedness in the physical and unpretentious bodies. The individual is a little molecule in the gigantic general field. A cognizant individual who knows about the unity of the fiery fields is freed from the deception that there is only a physical world in presence. Truth be told, each person is in real touch with the universe. In any case, as a result of issue and screw up, occurring in his very own vigorous fields, the awareness of man is obscured for a long spell of time. Therefore, he overlooks his sentiment of solidarity with God. The vast majority are not cognizant that a lively issue exists at the base of each physical issue. So as to treat the issue, we should change the quality and measure of vitality, which streams in the vivacious frameworks.

Our frame of mind to life impacts the manners in which we adapt to issues, both physical and mental the same. On the off chance that we live in agreement with the inestimable laws, we can be sound. Each dis-ease carries alongside it a message and a chance to learn and realize ourselves better. We should not fear from attempting to alter what is to be corrected. That is the reason each illness is in a manner our very own reflection inside states. Contamination of the blood as come about because of eating handled sustenance's, breathing unclean air and introduction to stress conditions are additionally at the foundation of our sicknesses.

Malady is a biochemical and electromagnetic dis-request of the cells in the body. It is brought about by negative feelings and it is a side effect of protection from change. The treatment of the indication alone doesn't fix the malady, on the grounds that there is a more profound reason for the ailment. Illnesses are the body's preliminary to dispose of toxin. This is the motivation behind why it is great to give the side effect a chance to convey what needs be drastically. We should experience the manifestation, with no emotional judgment or any displeasure. We should treat it with self-examination and with the information of the progression of vitality in the body. In the event that the parity in some part has been irritated, the entire living being is influenced right away.

Wellbeing is in actuality a declaration of the concordance between various types of energies. The healer transmits an electromagnetic charge that balance, arranges off toxic substances and brings wellbeing. A healer and a sound man have an excess of Prana - the inconspicuous vitality in charge of the body imperativeness, while a wiped out man is in a territory of Prana shortage.

There are a few phases in mending:

1. Checking if the treated patient gets the mending vitality with euphoria.
2. Diagnosing the quality.
3. Refining the emanation.
4. Transmitting vitality, from the healer to the treated patient.

5. Treating the Chakras, the meridians and adjusting the vitality.

The significance of profound breathing and a casual state are fundamental during the transmission of the recuperating vitality. With right gave individuals the left hand as a rule gets the vitality - for the most part the healer lifts the left hand upward to get infinite vitality. The dynamic right hand emanates the vitality and accordingly he holds it toward the patient air or the treated organ. With left-gave individuals, the activity is a remarkable inverse. Vitality may be gotten, coordinated or transmitted likewise through two hands. Mending can be constrained by the desire of the healer by means of idea and the healer can send vitality with two hands.

The extraction of foul vitality just as expansion of filtered vitality - delivers mending. The reason for some infections is an absence of vitality. Where there is a deterrent, there is additionally an amassing of vitality, an obstacle of the stream and that hindrance must be discharged. The healer ought to consistently have the patient's affirmation to treat him. The best perspective to transmit and get vitality is the point at which the mind conveys Alpha waves - the condition of unwinding. The healer must be in a condition of congruity with the patient, so as to transmit vitality proficiently.

There is no utilization in the transmission of vitality before refinement of the emanation. Electricity produced via friction, which holds fast to the atmosphere, averts the attainability of vitality transmission. This is the motivation behind why the quality is constantly cleansed before any transmission of vitality. In treating certain organ, or a specific spot in the body, it ought to be first cleansed. Filtration much of the time makes a nice sentiment. New age prescription uses vibration methods. At the point when these procedures are consolidated they increment gigantically the power of the vitality.

# CHAPTER EIGHT

## EXTRA TECHNIQUES TO USE WITH REIKI: CRYSTALS, MEDITATION, YOGA

### CRYSTALS

Gems have a sorted out geometric course of action of the molecules and in view of their organized structure they are in a condition of flawlessness. They transmit a solid rational vitality, which reverberates with the existence power. They have vitality fields, which impact man's electromagnetic field and can store different recollections. In the event that they stay in an unclean domain, their fiery recollections become hazardous as they emanate the negative vitality that was put away inside them. Precious stones can change the cerebrum waves on the off chance that they are put on a vitality focus - a reality confirmed with an Encephalogram instrument. On the off chance that they are set on needle therapy focuses, the skin obstruction changes, which demonstrates their capacity to change electric charges.

Precious stones have the property of engrossing electromagnetic vitality, store it, change it and discharge it. They likewise can stimulate body and soul. They make negative particles that reinforce the vitality of the body. The utilization of brilliant gems and precious stones is thusly suggested. Continuously spotless the gems before use, by absorbing them for one hour a blend of half liter of water, a spoon of ocean salt and a spoon of juice vinegar.

In performing treatment with gems, our mentality towards the gems is significant. Sending it our affection and having confidence in its beneficial outcome is significant. Use Jasper stone or a Tiger-eye stone to expand your vitality. Request that the precious stone improve your vitality, while holding it in your left getting hand. If there should be an occurrence of strain the vast majority utilize the

Aquamarine precious stone. The dark Tourmaline and Amber are fit for engrossing the body's cynicism. Each precious stone works in an alternate way. It is conceivable to increase the pace of vibration at home and kill negative impacts by setting gems at the sides of the rooms - quartz or Amethyst groups. In "Atlantis", the lost mainland a gem was introduced in each house and its capacity was to refine the air. Individuals in Atlantis utilized precious stones to improve the sun's vitality, they didn't need fuel.

Wearing a precious stone around our neck enacts the thymus organ and the invulnerability framework. It ought to be underlined however, that the precious stone increases the vibration it gets numerous falls. On the off chance that somebody is irate, the gem will build his resentment. While wearing the precious stone or utilizing it you ought to make sure to be in condition of affection and empathy so the gem will expand these positive characteristics.

Each gem has its specific trademark, Ruby influences love; Jade influences intelligence. Individuals are pulled in to gems due to their exceptional attributes.

Gems and precious stones encapsulate enormous forces, offering them to the individuals who wear them. Be that as it may, albeit valuable stones and precious stones may pass on their qualities, one ought not depend on only them. They won't "carry out the responsibility" for us. They are fit for moving astronomical vitality to us and we can utilize them similarly as an instrument to support us. On the off chance that we wish to make progress with precious stones, they ought to turn out to be a piece of us - some portion of our internal life. It isn't sufficient just to wear them, it is great to see them every now and then and fuse their qualities in us. Individuals are pulled in to them since they get and transmit the light.

While cooked, sustenance loses energy. In the event that we place nourishment on a precious stone board, we add vitality to it. Stone containing iron oxide or a quartz precious stone, one and half inch long in a liter of water during the night - improve the trial of the water and twofold its vitality. It is great to put gems or red hued stones in pockets, in work area drawers and in organizers. They add vitality to fabrics and cloth, while being put away. Precious stone sheets under a bundle of roses can extend the bloom's life. Precious stones lessen torment, recuperate the body and diminish physical and mental pressure. As of now referenced gems store and transmit vitality. Thought itself is vitality and we can program a precious stone and introduce an idea or a thought into it, and the gem thusly can fortify it and transmit it. That is the reason precious stones are utilized as a helping instrument in clairvoyance, reflection and recuperating.

Programming a precious stone – gems can be modified to help us. Above all else, you need to send love to the precious stone, hold it near your heart until you feel its closeness. Later on spot it on your temple, where the Third eye should be. Find in your creative mind the activity that the gem needs to accomplish for you, and envision that your contemplations are entering the gem. Its activity is subject to your capacity to focus and all alone contact with it. Thank the precious stone consistently, for its fruitful activity and find in your creative mind how the final product is accomplished. In the event that someone contacts the precious stone, it is important to purge it with water and ocean salt and modified once more. The purifying of the gem is done likewise by consuming incense of cedar and salvia.

Contemplation with a precious stone - plunk down restful with a straight back, holding the gem in the getting hand, the correct hand with a great many people. Watch the precious stone and reach it through your heart. Attempt to relate to it, gradually, gradually. Close your eyes and attempt to believe, to detect the precious stone with every one of its qualities - its temperature, its edges, its sentiments and its shading. It is critical to open up to the gem's vitality, which you can feel like warmth, cold or a jerk, and empower the vitality to scatter in your entire body. Envision that you are the gem that turns straightforward increasingly more in each passing minute, gets data from the earth and draws in magnificence, harmony and serenity.

Adjusting the two cerebrum sides of the equator with precious stones it is conceivable to adjust the two mind's sides of the equator with the guide of gems. Grasp a twofold ended precious stone and being in a reflective state, breathe in air in your lungs. Breathe out gradually, amass in your correct mind's side of the equator and close your left hand. Breathe in yet again, and keeping in mind that breathing out focus to your left side cerebrum's side of the equator - shutting your correct hand. Rehash this activity a few times. Taking care of issues with the guide of precious stones - If you feel anxious, it is great to hold a smoky quartz gem, to contact the earth with it and unwind. Later on you should hold a straightforward precious stone with two hands, announce so anyone might hear your concern, in a raised voice - attempting to consolidate your concern into the gem. You should consolidate the issue in the precious stone and after that clean the gem from its vibration in water and ocean salt. Toss the water with the gem's vibration into the ground and envision that there it is changed. This activity is utilized as a helper apparatus to take care of your concern, by accelerating the cognizant and the intuitive to act.

Recuperating with gems - Use precious stones as a helper apparatus in playing out the treatment of breathing, sounds and hues. Quartz (SiO2) is found in the body's cells, and influences them, as its vitality fields and vibration coordinate our own. In the event that you need to utilize a precious stone for self-recuperating: unwind in a helpful sitting position, or in lying position. Focus on the infected organ, the hurt spot and spot a precious stone on that spot or hold it in a natural way. You may utilize one precious stone or a blend of two gems or a few gems. Normally it is prescribed to use at any rate two quartz gems, with one end, and a length of at any rate two inches each. One is held in the left hand pointing towards the impact point of the hand, the other one in the correct hand, with its end coordinated towards the fingers. This situation of the precious stones enables the vitality to stream, considering that the correct hand emanates, while the left hand is getting. From the outset you simply envision the progression of vitality, however after some time, you will feel the progression of vitality, spilling in your body and the infected organ.

Gems impact monstrously the vitality focuses. Red and orange gems are utilized to reinforce the essentialness, blue and green gems to re-establish the body and violet stones are utilized for otherworldly improvement. It is prescribed to put the precious stones and gems with the correct shading, on the different vitality focuses: blue on the throat, green on the heart. Something very similar works when we put them on our photo, or the photo of somebody we wish to fix. The photo has a similar vibration of the man envisioned in it. The technique works great. It is great to check with a pendulum the period of time the precious stones should remain on the photo.

A Quartz gem on the Root's chakra brings a sentiment of confidence, into our day by day life. A Quartz precious stone on the Sexual chakra encourages us in sexual connections and brings essentialness. On the Solar plexus it illuminates our character. A man, who looks for places of intensity for himself, must offset the Solar plexus with philanthropy - the thought of other individuals' prosperity. A Quartz gem set on the Heart chakra purges our affection and increases our internal power. On Throat chakra it delivers expert articulation and clearness to our discourse. On the

6th chakra, it clears our considerations, balances the two mind halves of the globe and upgrades the power over the psychological body. Set on the seventh chakra, the precious stone upgrades correspondence with the profound world and encourages the individual sense of self to join with the "Higher Self". A Quartz precious stone put on a chakra with its honed end towards our head filters the chakra. The amethyst stone frees us from material reliance and gets in touch with us with our imaginative forces. Amethyst stones, set on each chakra in the body, and one between the legs, help to connect with the Soul. Sapphires guarantee peacefulness and serenity and fortify our confidence.

Sea green/blue stones empower us to increase our mending power. With the help of seven Rose quartz stones we can get closer to the best righteousness - to unequivocal love. Garnet stones bring bliss and vitality, and Amber stones bring achievement. In the event that you wish to get recuperating vitality inside 24 hours, place your or another person photo (if a photo is inaccessible, you may put hair or much finger-nails rather) on a level quartz or Agate board, on which you have included little green gems, in the state of a Star of David and a gem in the Star of David.

Pink and Green precious stones are utilized for affection; violet gems are utilized for otherworldliness. Gems are wellspring of vitality and excellence and are utilized for: 1) Healing. 2) Massaging the reflex focuses in the body, legs and hands. 3) Treating suitable needle therapy focuses (with a Quartz precious stone three times each day). 4) Water, in which you place a gem for three hours, is useful for drinking and can be utilized for getting ready wet gauzes, or for a shower. 5) Crystals put on vitality focuses – help to open up blockages and are a guide for profound improvement. 6) To adjust the chakras, place the seven gems that have a place with the chakras (see the outlines at the section of the chakras) in a straightforward glass in the sun during the day, and in the moon light during the night. Drink a spoonful of water once per day. 7) Crystals are utilized as a special necklace. Wear them on the body, on the materials, or put them even underneath the pad. 8) You may put them on all aspects of the body that needs to experience an activity, before the activity and after it. The precious stone's attributes are subject to their synthesis, size, virtue, shape and shading. In this manner a watermelon Tourmaline is amazing for the Heart chakra, a pink Tourmaline fortifies the capacity of insight, a green Tourmaline sedates and dark Tourmaline grounds us and shields us from negative vibrations.

The following are the characteristics of some of the crystals:

Straightforward Quartz - purges, expands the faculties and blesses all the unpretentious bodies with vitality.

Precious stones and straightforward Quartz are vitality intensifiers.

Garnet - fortifies the body, the blood, and is utilized against torments, discouragement and apprehensive depletion.

Lapis Lazuli - builds mental power. It is productive for the throat vitality focus, helps clear self-expression in discourse, expands fearlessness and improves rest.

Lazurit - loosens up the muscles. It is useful for torn ligaments, for stomach and back issues.

Malachite - can draw out agony and it is prescribed for blood treatment, the liver, nerve bladder, hurting joints and stiffness.

Ruby - is suggested for stomach, belly and entrail issues, and wipes out toxic substances.

Opal - is being utilized against looseness of the bowels and against a sleeping disorder (by putting it underneath the cushion).

Amethyst - sedates and it is utilized against a sleeping disorder, thyroid issue and for profound elevating.

Obsidian and calcite - treat bones, inclined to breaking for absence of calcium, anticipate osteoporosis.

Citrine - is a tissue regenerator, purifying, growing and adjusting the vitality of the body and the emanation.

Topaz - accelerates moderate working organs, accelerates vitality focuses and discharges adrenaline into the blood. It is utilized against a sleeping disorder, depletion and thrombosis.

Kunzite - purifies antagonism, bringing equalization and steadiness.

Jade - stimulates the blood flow, the mind's activity, is nerve - reinforcing and is useful for the heart, liver and kidneys.

Magnetite - emanates attractive vitality, captivates the Yin and Yang energies.

Moldavit - rises vibrations and illuminates the spirit.

Tektite and Boji stones - adjusts, balances out and cleans the whole atmosphere and the chakras frameworks.

To cause a buzz of quietness and harmony utilize a Sapphire. Lapis Lazuli and Tourmaline widen the awareness. Quartz and Meteorite help to create inestimable awareness, Tourmaline bolster representation.

Precious stone and Beryl bolster clairvoyance, Hekimar jewel and Opal are utilized for knowledge and perceptiveness, topaz for internal quality and Jade for insight.

## MEDICATION

Medication is a procedure through which you can experience quietness and a peaceful personality. The Reiki thoughtful vitality is recuperating and cherishing. It includes images and mantras to encourage your contemplation experience. It positions high among the conventional recuperating frameworks. Look at beneath to discover the way of its training. As vitality is moved, mending can happen; and Reiki contemplation strategy can help this procedure along. Specialists of this sort of contemplation can mend others and even themselves by diverting Reiki's recuperating energy. The patient's vitality field is adjusted and everything will be in agreement once more.

The homeostasis is simply the body's normal equalization, and submerging in Reiki Meditation can enable you to accomplish impeccable parity. The body's needs vitality to recuperate, and through this reflection that vitality can really originate from other individuals. There are various mending systems that are consolidated together to frame Reiki Meditation. It has been built up that the underlying foundations of contemplation originate from the Vedic age. The Vedic individuals used to rehearse these strategies to mollify their divine beings, which they used to dread and love. There has been some discussion on its reality before the Vedic age too. In different ancient human advancements there have been hints of these systems being utilized to connect with the maker of this world, by redundantly reciting certain musical melodies.

This routine with regards to interacting with your cognizance is a delightful inclination. Day by day rehearsing these techniques makes you flawless and quiets your psyche, body and soul. Today our everyday lives are loaded with weights, duties and bedlam. There is no space for reflection and contemplation. The tension builds so much that individuals get discouraged, pushed and disturbed effectively. You will seldom run over an individual who is by all accounts glad and isn't experiencing pressure. By rehearsing reflection, you can explore through every one of these issues.

## Eight Ancient Guided Medication Techniques to Know!

These 8 antiquated methods have been around for more than a huge number of years and have stood the trial of time. Seeing every reflection procedure will give you a diagram of the aim and reason for the apparatus to enable any fledglings to move beyond the underlying obstacles to realize inward harmony inside, while simultaneously discharge worry to advance recuperating for the psyche and body.

The old yogic experts knew a huge number of years before that our bodies are not only material in nature. They are additionally certainly enthusiastic in nature. Science has amassed impressive learning concerning this electromagnetic, bioenergetics working of the human body.

In any case, researchers are first to concede that they don't generally fathom the hidden powers that create life. Logical instruments can look just so far into the issue vitality continuum before arriving at their perceptual points of confinement. The extraordinary thing about reflection is that there's nobody size-fits-all arrangement. A few people ponder by sitting unobtrusively in the solace of their home, while others may state that their yoga practice fills in as their reflection. In any case which strategy is utilized, the objective is consistently the equivalent, discover what impacts you and supports you in your development.

1) Guided reflection

Guided reflection is a mix of mesmerizing and representation. It isn't exemplary reflection since it depends on outside improvements, however it is only a stage away from it. The style it uses shifts as it takes the person on an adventure of the faculties and psyche to advance unwinding.

2) Chakra contemplation

Chakras are a Sanskrit word that implies vortexes of vitality. These are essentially vitality zones in our body. There are seven fundamental vortexes and they control various parts of our human and otherworldly lives. A few conventions perceive that, from the medicinal term of the physical body, this seven vitality focuses are viewed as the endocrine framework.

3) Kundalini reflection

Kundalini, which in Sanskrit is followed to the word kundala (which signifies "wound"), over ages came to allude to the inert intensity of profound acknowledgment covered where it counts in the human body, interminably compelled to ascend and show its definitive certainties, power, and rapture. There is a connection among Kundalini and the seven chakra vitality.

4) Mantra contemplation

Mantra reiteration just means rehashing a sentence or gathering of words that have a phonetic noteworthiness. Mantra is inherently identified with sound. Mantra is sound, and sound is resonating in everything in this universe. Present day researchers are starting to perceive as our old sages did, that there exists a vibration which resonates incessantly all through the universe. Models are the sound 'Om' or 'Aum' or even 'I am that I am'.

5) Reiki reflection

Reiki (articulated beam key) is a characteristic recuperating procedure that feels like a progression of a high recurrence of vitality into and through a specialist, and out the hands into someone else. For all intents and purposes anybody can learn Reiki with no related knowledge or capacity important. The attunement procedure opens the heart, crown and palm chakras and makes an exceptional connection between the understudy and the Reiki source.

6) Mindfulness reflection

Care is a capacity to focus with a specific goal in mind, deliberately and purpose, focused right now and relinquishing decisions. A few activities that include the training are standing contemplation, strolling reflection or eating contemplation. The thought stems from this thought "Any place You Go, Whatever You Do, and There You Are"!

7) Pyramid contemplation

Pyramid contemplation may have been gotten from the antiquated Egyptians, they utilized pyramids as graves and sanctuaries however they additionally utilized them as approaches to ground and change over vast energies. In the present current world, there are reflection pyramid structures that can be acquired or one can be worked at home by simply utilizing bits of wood and pondering inside.

8) Qigong contemplation

Kenneth Cohen deciphers Qigong as "working with life vitality, figuring out how to control the stream and dispersion of qi to improve the wellbeing and congruity of psyche and body." Such practices have been pervasive in China for 2000-3000 years. The focal thought in qigong practice is the control and control of qi, a type of vitality.

**The Reiki Meditation Technique**

Purging the System

Chakra Forces

Recuperating through Hands

Last thought

## 1. Purging The System

Plunk down or rests serenely on a tangle with your back straight. Attempt to be quiet, made, and loose. Take a full breath. Envision yourself breathing in all the joy and goodness that you need, and breathing out profoundly with the idea that negative feelings, for example, despondency, dread, and tension, are being flushed out of your framework. Inhale two or multiple times thusly, and see how your psyche and body tune into it and unwind.

## 2. Chakra Forces

There are seven chakras in your body, from the base of your spine to the highest point of your head, which are vitality focuses of the body. Spot your turn before your body at each chakra zone and hold at each situation for a couple of minutes, contingent upon your body's need. In the event that you feel your body is requesting the hand to remain for a more drawn out time, let it remain. Evacuate it if your body has had enough. Feeling through the hands is the most ideal approach to interface and tune in to your body. As you tune into your body through your hands, envision the existence power of the universe entering your body through your hands, with the chakras as the mode of entry. Feel your body resound with this vitality stream, and go into a condition of profound unwinding and restoration.

## 3. Recuperating Through Hands

To begin with, place your palms together over your head. Hold the hands there and attempt to tune in to your body with consideration and consideration. At the same time, inhale profoundly and gradually, expelling the negatives and soaking up the positives into your framework. Unwind. Spot your hands on the temple and after that at the back of your head. Next, go down to the throat and put one hand tenderly on it and the other on the back of your neck. Hold it for quite a while and unwind.

Presently, go down and place your hands on the back of your shoulders, with the fingers looking down, on your chest covering your heart, on the lower chest close to the ribs, on your stomach, and after that the lower mid-region. Ensure that at each position, you are delicate with your touch. Hold the hand till your body requests it, unwind and move to the following part.

In the wake of completing the head and middle, go down to your hips and spot your hands on both your hips, the knees, and the feet. For the feet, put your hands either over them or the base contingent upon your comfort. At every crossroads, feel the vitality course through your body. Appreciate the experience.

## 4. Last Thought

Recover your hands in the petition position and spot them before your chest. Sit with your spine straight and your body marginally tight. Inhale regularly and feel the vitality going through your body. Do this for around 3-5 minutes or till you want to do it. The recuperating procedure is finished when you feel lighted and empowered.

You will have the option to recuperate normally, and improve your body and brain through this straightforward and loosening up system. When you can associate your soul to your body, you will discover numerous medications and treatments are essentially progressively successful. Reiki Masters show the craft of Reiki Meditation, and understudies think that its extremely simple to learn. You will appreciate a ton of medical advantages when you play out this sort of reflection.

**Advantages of Reiki Meditation**

- Reiki reflection will loosen up your psyche and lessen pressure
- It will give reliable
- The reflection builds your discernment and representation
- It raises your cognizance and betters your capacity to tackle issues
- This system is generally known to fix numerous illnesses

- It is perfect for post-medical procedure mending
- It helps great rest
- Reiki contemplation functions admirably with other mending/medicinal procedures
- This system expels vitality hinders in your body, empowering free vitality stream, which gives you a solid body
- It is a self-improvement and change device

## YOGA

Practice yoga and be the best surfer that you can be. Each genuine surfer needs to keep up a solid and dapper body and furthermore a quiet demeanour when taking part in such testing game. Surfing educators and specialists state that it's significant not exclusively to be physically adaptable, adjusted and not effectively exhausted, yet in addition to be rationally arranged. Yoga can do much in giving the stamina and mental moulding for surfing.

You may rehearse yoga in various ways. You can try out a class directly in the city and get familiar with the essential yoga aptitudes that can quiet the faculties and improve stance and relaxing. Or on the other hand you can cruise away to an intriguing goal on the off chance that you have the cash and appreciate a reviving bundle that incorporates yoga, knead, nature climbing, and surfing. Yoga styles differ. A few organizations consolidate the different standards to enable people to have a more grounded, more beneficial and increasingly mollified stream. Individuals leave from a yoga class feeling less focused and on edge and prepared to receive the rewards of a life that is increasingly adjusted.

The intensity of the sea can be overpowering; however, a surfer can remain in direction with legitimate personality moulding for surfing. When you've left on a daring, thrilling get-away and you've enrolled the administrations of a group of specialists to help give an all-encompassing background that incorporates yoga and surfing, you can carry your surfing to the following level.

For apprentices, yoga can be rehearsed a very long time ahead of time before trekking to a surfing spot. By helping increment parity, dependability, and power, the mind-loosening up action can give you a chance to skim with less exertion and stretch yourself as far as possible with less spills.

Surfing's a game that involves extraordinary physical effort. You need impeccable planning and settle on split-second choices as a wave draws near. In case you're simply beginning, your appendages will throb and you'll be winded after so much paddling and adjusting. The weariness might be sufficient to make the normal individual surrender. A reviving yoga class or loosening up system like Reiki in the wake of surfing can facilitate the pressure and offer profound unwinding.

A yoga ace may direct you through planned activities like 20 minutes of focused postures for the abs and back, about thirty minutes of improving mental center, and a couple of minutes of a loosening up succession to evacuate pressure and impart quiet vitality. Through remedial exemplary yoga, you can make a brain, body and soul association and get recharged moulding for surfing. Most surf and yoga bundles offered by picturesque goals off the beaten track offer solid natural dinners to go with a paramount surfing background and get-away.

One of the most generally rehearsed types of yoga is asana, or stances that interface development with breath. Be that as it may, there is significantly more about yoga to investigate past asana; seven different appendages, truth be told. There may come a period in your training where physical postures aren't as basic as what is sprouting inside.

## Reiki and Yoga Together

Yoga and Reiki can be utilized related to each other to encounter extreme change. Yoga can be compared to stripping ceaselessly the layers of an onion. As each layer sheds, increasingly more disentangles about oneself. The procedure can be both enabling and somewhat unnerving.

It is between these touchy layers where the use of vitality work, for example, Reiki can have an extraordinary reaction. When one is totally open to accepting, Reiki will go to the zone of the body, psyche, or soul, where it is generally required. During a workshop I was holding, one understudy felt a profound association with a misfortune that the individual by him was encountering, however the individual hadn't imparted this data to the gathering. The understudy had the option to connect and offer unequivocal love and comprehension.

In another example, an understudy got the bump to leave the vocation way she was as of now on and roll out an improvement.

Planning for Healing

To plan to mend with both yoga and Reiki, first supplant uncertainty and dread with a feeling of experience!

Start with moderate, deliberate breath and contemplation before starting asana. Your asana practice can last from a couple of minutes up to a full yoga practice. After development, locate an upheld seat or leaned back posture, for example, Savasana to start a self-treatment, or have a Reiki expert encourage mending.

Keep an open heart, and discharge any connection to the result of your session. In spite of the fact that

Reiki and yoga are altogether different, rehearsing them together can be a lucky disclosure for feeding the internal identity.

# CONCLUSION

For our very own wellbeing, it is essential to breath appropriately (energy retention through breathing), to eat well nourishment (ingestion of vitality from sustenance) and live in a vivacious area where there is no fiery vacuum. It is prescribed to treat illnesses before their appearance in the physical body, for the correct capacity of the vivacious frameworks of the body. At the point when malady shows up, it is essential to comprehend what the infection is attempting to let us know and to treat it in a vivacious way - notwithstanding ordinary treatment.

The body, the air, and the chakras, bring to mind a dark opening, which ingests the encompassing vitality. They get data as vitality from the earth, process it as indicated by the person's degree of improvement, and emanate it back to the earth. The spirit is the endless eyewitness, who perspectives beneficial encounters and gets intelligence from life tests. In the event that we stay in contact with the spirit, we know who we truly are, and thusly we can carry on agreeing the desire of the spirit, which is unlimited love and satisfaction. We arrive at the element of the spirit, in the event that we filter our character, open our hearts, and coordinate the two halves of the globe of the minds. We ought to do a profound and inside change that would cleanse the cognizant and intuitive mindfulness from injury and negative musings and sentiments. At exactly that point, we can construct the collection of light - the physical body, the atmosphere, and the chakras will be flooded with light. At exactly that point, we can wind up solid and progress while in transit to illumination.

There are three different ways, in which we can work, for the rebuilding of our wellbeing and our otherworldly improvement:

1. Purging of the quality, the cognizant and intuitive contemplations and emotions. When us

2. atmosphere in sanitized we become the vessel of the Will of God.

3.  Appropriate treatment of the progression of vitality in the meridians. Dread, negative sentiments, ceaseless pressure hinder the progression of vitality in the meridians.

4.  Improvement of the energy focuses in the entirety of their measurements. Adjusted advancement of the energy focuses is imperative for wellbeing and will acquire its wake, disposal of inward logical inconsistencies and extension of cognizance. We will have the option to appreciate the universe of duality when we understand that our self-esteem isn't relying upon winning or losing or on being male or female.

In the vitality framework, each passionate and mental issue is communicated. An enthusiastic change is first communicated in the quality, in the meridians and in the chakras and just later it is found in the physical body. The mystery of recuperating is parity and congruity. The body's wellbeing is significant for our profound improvement. Be that as it may, the strength of the physical body is likewise associated with the wellbeing of the unobtrusive bodies and the association of Man with his spirit.

Dear readers, you have found out about the interior changes of the vigorous frameworks in the person. Presently you are set up to improve your very own life. Ask yourselves - what is your physical state, what is your passionate and mental state, and what do your spirit needs. Approach yourself what would you be able to accomplish for your own advantage, and how you can profit your fellowmen and your condition? With welcome of Light, improvement and wellbeing.